WHAT WOULD
HIPPOCRATES SAY?

WHAT WOULD HIPPOCRATES SAY?

Ancient Wisdom for Health, Fitness, and Fat Loss

JACOB
CALDWELL

Also by Jacob Caldwell

Images of Vitality: Reimagining Eating and Exercising

Poems for Vitality: An Education by Metaphor

Tending the Body: The Subtleness of Suppleness

Table of Contents

List of Abbreviations for Works Cited

Culpepper: Culpeper. *Complete Herbal & English Physician*. Manchester: J. Gleave and Son, 1826.

Dioscorides: Dioscorides. *Herbal*.

Art: Galen. *Art of Physick*. Trans. Nicholas Culpeper.

Hygiene: Galen. *Hygiene*. Trans. Robert Montraville Green. Springfield: Charles C Thomas, 1951.

Food: Galen. *On Food and Diet*. Trans. Mark Grant. London: Routledge, 2000.

Selected: Galen. *Selected Works*. Trans. P. N. Singer. New York: Oxford University Press, 1997.

Grieve: Grieve. *A Modern Herbal*. Stone Basin Books, 1931.

Hippocrates 1: Loeb Classical Library. *Hippocrates*. Volume I. Trans. W. H. S. Jones. (1: Ancient Medicine, Airs, Epidemics, Precepts, Nutriment).

Hippocrates 4: Loeb Classical Library. *Hippocrates*. Volume 4. Trans. W. H. S. Jones.

In honor of our Western heritage:
Thousands of years dedicated to the care for the body.

"... health precedes disease, so we ought to consider first how health may be preserved...."[1]

---

1 Hygiene. P5.

Introduction

*"Foolish the doctor who despises knowledge acquired
by the ancients." - Hippocrates*

Imagine being healthy, never being sick, always being
comfortable. Imagine a life without aches and pains. Imagine
having a strong, active body; a trim, lean figure. The ancient
Greeks knew that diet and exercise were the keys to health,
and they have much to teach us about such practices. The
ancient art of hygiene, the balancing of the body so as to gain
and maintain health, is a 2500 year old tradition. These are
the things that Hippocrates, the Father of Medicine writing in
the 400s BC, tells us how to do. In this book, we'll explore the
ancient tradition of Western health practices by asking the
question: what would Hippocrates say? What would
Hippocrates tell us if we asked him how to be healthy?

In order to answer this question, we need to start by
imagining our bodies the way he imagined the body. The
flesh of our bodies is made of the earth, and the life force
within us is a flame that burns within our flesh. We hold within
us the flame of life, and we melt the flesh of our bodies with
each passing second. We are born with only so much heat
and with only so much flesh. Both must be tended. We must
eat food to restock our flesh so that the fire of life has
something to burn, and we must exercise by living active lives

in order to kindle the flame of life. Even though we replenish our bodies with eating and even though we fan the flame with exercise, the process of replenishment is not perfect, and it does not last forever. The flame slowly wanes cold. The moisture of our flesh eventually dries up. Eventually we grow cold and dry, and when the heat and the moisture are gone, we die.

This image of life as a flame which consumes its moisture, of heat growing cold but being kindled by exercise, and of moisture drying out but being maintained by eating, is the ancient way of imagining how the body functions. It was the way that Hippocrates, the ancient Greek physician and the Father of Medicine, imagined things, and it was the way that Galen, the famous Roman doctor, did too. It was the guiding mythology of ancient medicine. We use the word 'mythology' here not in a derogatory sense, but in the sense of a story that helped to make sense of the art of medicine. It was the theory behind the practice. This mythology is the way Hippocrates and Galen, and many other physicians of ancient times, imagined things to be, and it helped to organize their thinking and actions. As we shall discuss in the pages of this book, this ancient way of imagining how the body functions proves to be extremely useful. It will help us to reimagine the concept of health, and it will help guide us to make healthy decisions.

This is a book about health, and the word 'health' comes from a Germanic word which means 'whole.' Being healthy is about being whole. To the ancient mind, to be whole was to have one's flame burning strongly, and to have plenty of good moisture for it to burn. Health, or wholeness, is about having the right amount of heat and the right amount of moisture. But as we shall see, too much of a good thing is not a good thing at all. The key to health is to have everything in proper balance.

We need to gain a deeper understanding of this ancient mythology of health if we are to be able to make good use of it. The basic idea is that our bodies are made of a mixture of heat, coldness, moisture, and dryness. Too much of any of these things is what causes disease. If we have too much heat, then we'll not only burn up, but the heat will also dry us out. We'll be charred crisps. On the other hand, if we have an excess of cold, then we won't be able to keep the flame of life going, and we'll get overloaded with moisture because there won't be enough heat to keep us reasonably dry. The same is true of too much moisture and of too much dryness: too much or too little of anything leads to problems. The key is to balance each of the four forces: to be hot but not too hot, cold but not too cold, wet but not too wet, and dry but not too dry.

Health is balance, and the word 'balance' really is the key word for health. The word 'balance' comes from the Latin 'bi-' meaning 'two' and 'lanx' meaning 'scalepan.' The word literally means 'having two scalepans.' In other words, to balance is to evenly distribute two things. If we could extend this to four things, that of heat, cold, moisture, and dryness, then it would be the perfect word for our purposes. Perhaps 'quadlanx' should be our term, but for simplicity's sake we will stick with the word 'balance.' Galen expresses the fantasy of balanced health quite nicely in the following quote:

> According to our standards, the ideal body weight is midway between thin and [obese].... And likewise of the other extremes, the ideal is such that one could not call it either hirsute or bald, soft or hard, white or black, large-veined or small-veined, irascible or serene, drowsy or wakeful, sluggish or alert, voluptuous or frigid. And if the exact mean of all the extremes were in all parts of the body, this would be the best to observe as being the symmetry most suitable for all activities.[2]

A useful image for this ancient idea of health is that we each must balance on a wobble board. Imagine a circular board with a rounded bottom on which one must stand. The front of the board is coldness. The back of the board is heat. The right side is moisture, and the left side is dryness. As we attempt to balance on this board, if we tilt too far in any direction, then we end up getting some form of disease. If we topple backward into heat, then we may end up with heartburn. If we fall rightward into excessive moisture, then we may end up with diarrhea. The idea is to stay balanced at all times.

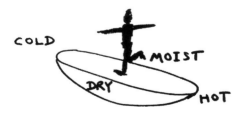

---

2   Hygiene. Book 1, Chapter 6.

Life is a constant challenge to our balance. As we will discuss in detail, the weather presents us with heat, cold, dryness, and moisture, in varying degrees throughout the year. As we age, we grow dryer and colder. We are each born with different propensities, some easily becoming hot; others cold, dry, or wet. And our actions in life can heat us, cool us down, dry us out, or drown us in moisture. Life knocks us around, and it is our job to stay balanced on the wobble board. A healthy person is someone who keeps him- or herself balanced.

We are going to be learning from Hippocrates and Galen in this book. Many quotes from each of them will appear in these pages. They will serve as our teachers about health. Hippocrates is said to have been born in 460 BC. He is considered the Father of Medicine. His writings, many of which were not actually written by him but which have been attributed to him through the ages, form the beginnings of Western medical thought. They are full of ancient wisdom about health. Galen, Hippocrates' greatest admirer, was born in 131 AD. He was the physician for the Roman Emperor Marcus Aurelius. Galen championed the works of Hippocrates and expanded upon them, carrying on the tradition of ancient medicine. One of his books, entitled *Hygiene*, was written specifically to help people to become healthy and to stay healthy. Galen's *Hygiene* will be frequently quoted as we explore the ancient ideas of health.

In this book we'll be asking ourselves: What would Hippocrates say? It's the question Galen seems to have asked himself throughout his career as a physician. By asking such a question, we search for firm ground on which to place our feet, a rock upon which to stand that carries the authority of our ancestors and the weight of history. It's the key question for our health: what would Hippocrates, the hero of the ancient art of health, say to us if we were to ask him about our health? If we were to ask Hippocrates how we could live healthier lives, what would he say? That's what this book tries to answer.

It's important to note that we are not literally asking Hippocrates this question. He is long-dead, many of his writings were not even written by him, and he wrote so long ago that his writings cannot possibly speak to the exact needs of today. Instead we are using Hippocrates as an imaginary figure to guide us. We hope to speak with his force, with his character, with his essence. It is his image that we seek to find in this book. Galen seems to be Hippocrates reborn, a man of similar disposition and calling. We ask for their imaginary answers to our questions about health.

What Hippocrates has to say will prove to be very useful. The ancient ideas about health really do work. The theory, though perhaps literally wrong, is imaginatively powerful, for it guides us into useful actions. The ancient ideas about health are a lot like Newton's laws of physics, which, after Einstein, are known to be literally incorrect, but they are every bit as useful as they ever were for everyday purposes. For all intents and purposes in our daily lives, gravity still pulls down toward the center of the earth, even though physicists now imagine space and time to be curved. It is likewise for the ancient concepts of health. When we imagine an excess of heat in our bodies, it's very easy to understand that we need to do something to cool it down. The images are very powerful, and they have an effect on our imaginations as well. It's amazing how quickly a sore throat reduces in intensity when it is imagined to be caused by excessive moisture oozing out of the head, and thus treated with herbs that will dry it. The herbs may have absolutely no actual, literal effect on the sore throat, but in the world of the imagination, the phlegm is dried, and the sore throat is soothed.

The ideas that we will be discussing in this book are ancient. They are extremely useful, and they carry a profound wisdom. But we must be careful not to take them too literally. The argument we will be making in this book is not that these ancient ideas are superior to our modern ideas. It isn't about who is right and who is wrong. It's about what is *useful*. The challenge for anyone reading this book is the challenge of being able to imagine things in multiple, sometimes conflicting ways. The next time we catch a cold and have thick snot dripping from the nose, we want to be able to imagine it as both a viral infection *and* an excess of rheum (which is what the ancients called this substance) in the head. Certainly modern medicine is correct in saying that a virus has entered the body. But that is not the only legitimate way of imagining what is happening. It is also true that, if the nose runs with thick yellow snot, then there is an excess of rheum in the head being purged through the nose. If we can't imagine the virus, then we can't do anything about it, such as washing our hands to keep from spreading the virus to others. In the same way, if we can't imagine the excess of rheum, then we can't do anything to manage it. Hippocrates would tell us that the rheum is excessive because the brain is too moist and needs to be dried. He would suggest certain drying herbs. Both the idea of the virus and the idea of the rheum are extremely useful in managing a thick, snotty nose. But we have to be able to imagine both if we want to be able to benefit from both. *Both* have merit. The modern mythology is useful, and so is the ancient mythology. The ancient mythology was actively used for thousands of years. The modern and the ancient don't have to compete with each other for which is 'right.' They can both be useful.

In order to benefit from the ancient wisdom of Hippocrates, we must be able to imagine things the way he imagined them. We must imagine our bodies as complex amalgams of heat, coldness, moisture, and dryness. We must imagine ourselves in need of constant balance. We stand upon the wobble board, striving to keep level.

Many of the ideas in this book will inspire us to make changes, to try out some seemingly new (though actually very old) concepts about health. But there is one major piece of ancient advice that we must bear in mind: health abhors sudden changes. Galen says that changes should "... be done by degrees, for nature abhors all sudden change,"[3] and Hippocrates says,

---

3   Art. Ch 86.

It is changes that are chiefly responsible for diseases, especially the greatest changes, the violent alterations both in the seasons and in other things. But seasons which come on gradually are the safest, as are gradual changes of regimen and temperature, and gradual changes from one period of life to another.[4]

If we are going to make a change, then we must make it a *gradual* change. If we're going to start eating a drier diet, then we should replace a few moistening foods with a few drying foods, not change everything all at once. Health does not result from going 'cold turkey'! Make it a slow, steady transition. If we make drastic changes, then we will end up getting hurt. Making slow changes is one of the first and primary rules of the wisdom of Hippocrates.

Perhaps the most important thing Hippocrates has to say to us is the following. We are each born with a certain constitution, with an individual propensity for heat or cold, dryness or moisture. As we age, our constitution changes. The world around us, most notably the seasons and the weather, add heat or coldness, dryness or moisture. All of these things affect us and make us more or less prone to disease. But we do not control our constitutions, we cannot stop aging, and we cannot control the weather. This leaves us seemingly defenseless. How can we balance ourselves if the world is just knocking us around without any way for us to regain our footing? The answer is that we are not as defenseless as it may seem. We do have control over our food and over our exercise, and therefore diet and exercise

---

4 Hippocrates 4, Humours, Ch 16.

are our primary means of attempting to balance. Hippocrates explains: "For food and exercise, while possessing opposite qualities, yet work together to produce health. For it is the nature of exercise to use up material, but of food and drink to make good deficiencies."[5] Diet and exercise are the ways that we can adjust ourselves on the wobble board of health. When life pushes us around, diet and exercise keep us from falling. The flip side of this is that diet and exercise can also make things much worse. They are powerful tools that we must learn to use for balance instead of imbalance.

In this book we will first discuss the things over which we have no control: the seasons, our constitutions, and aging. Then we will discuss how to recognize when we have been thrown off-balance by learning to recognize the signs of imbalance. Then we will discuss what we can do about imbalance by learning to use diet and exercise to balance ourselves. And finally, and most importantly, we will discuss how to make use of what Hippocrates says not just for health, but for living our lives with more vitality.

This book is a practical guide to ancient health practices. It is not about treating diseases, but about the ancient ideas of how to be healthy and stay healthy. It is about balancing the forces of life so that we can stay healthy and avoid the need for medical treatment. But of course, once we get a disease, we should not try to manage it on our own with the ideas in this book. This book does not substitute for real medical help.

---

5 Hippocrates 4, Regimen 1, Ch 2.

Instead, it is a way to reimagine the concept of health itself, and to become truly healthy and more vitally alive.

The Forces of Imbalance

"It is chiefly the changes of the seasons which produce disease, and in the seasons the great changes from cold to heat, and so on according to the same rule."[6] - Hippocrates

The quote above is striking. According to the Father of Medicine, the seasons are the primary cause of disease. Specifically, it is the *changes* that occur with the seasons that cause us problems. It is the change from hot to cold, cold to hot, dry to moist, and moist to dry, which are to blame for most illnesses. Galen says, "... the subject of airs, waters, and places... forms part of the first division of the art of caring...."[7] By this he means that one's environment is paramount to one's health. To ancient people, the weather was remarkably important.

When it's hot, heat is being added to our bodies. We are being pushed toward the hot side of the wobble board. In order to maintain our balance, we must lean toward the cold side of the board. The same is true with coldness, moisture, and dryness. Each season brings with it a new force in our lives. In general, spring is hot and moist, summer is hot and dry, autumn is cold and dry, and winter is cold and moist.

---

6 Hippocrates 4, Aphorisms, Book 3.
7 Selected. P90.

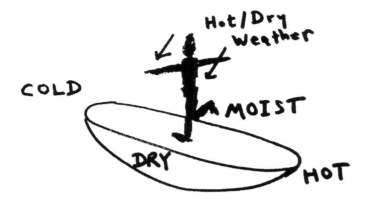

The influence of each season is quite logical when one thinks it through. It all hinges on the sun. In the deep of winter the world sees less of the warmth of the sun and is therefore cold, but also full of moisture, since the heat of the sun doesn't just warm but also dries things. In winter, when the sun is as weak as it ever gets, the world is as cold and as moist as it can be. So winter is cold and moist. As spring begins, the sun starts to warm the world again, but the moisture is not yet dried. So the spring is a time of heat and moisture. It is a warming transition toward the summer. When summer arrives and the sun is at its height of power, the moisture has been dried, leaving the world hot and dry for the summertime. Then, as autumn comes and the sun begins to fade, the world cools but is still left dry by summer. So autumn is cold and dry. And finally as winter returns and the sun further fades, the cold reaches its peak so that moisture is able to fully return, leaving winter cold and moist.

Of course, sometimes there is unseasonable weather. Sometimes it rains in August and sometimes there's a heatwave in January. And even more important, many places in the world are not at all dry in the summer, but very humid instead. They are hot and moist in the summer. In fact, some places are hot all year, such as the tropics. If one lives in the tropics, then one is almost constantly being pushed toward the hot side of the board. Conversely, in one lives in a very cold place, then one is probably being pushed toward the cold side of the board all year, even when it's relatively warm. The point is that we can't follow general guidelines in this process. Just because the textbook says that it's hot and dry in summer, that doesn't mean it's always hot and dry in summer, or even that it's hot and dry at all in a particular place and at a particular time. The key is to recognize what the weather is doing to us. If it's incredibly dry, our bodies react very dramatically. We can get thrown off-balance very easily by any major change in the weather, or by any prolonged weather pattern. The ancients recognized this important force in their lives, and took actions to balance it out.

We in this modern world need to realize that we very much manipulate our personal weather. Although it may be very cold and moist outside, perhaps even snowing, we may spend most of the winter being warmed and dried by a heater. We may actually be living in a hot and very dry environment even when it's cold and moist outside. So although the weather may be one way, we may in fact be affected by a dramatically different 'weather.' Both air conditioning and heaters dramatically change our personal 'weather.' In general, we in the modern world live in drier weather than we often realize. Those who use humidifiers have just the opposite situation. Their world is moister than the outside world. It's not that any of these technologies are unhealthy. We just need to recognize the 'weather' that they bring into our lives, and we need to recognize the force that may need balancing in order to maintain our health.

One of the major reasons that changes in weather are so challenging for health is that changes in weather bring changes in the forces affecting our ability to balance on the wobble board of health. If it has been cold lately and if we've been doing alright balancing on the board of health, then that means that we've been leaning at least slightly toward the hot side of the board in order to balance against the cold. But if the weather suddenly switches to hot, then we, already leaning toward the hot side of the board, can easily be thrown off-balance with the change in the weather. As the weather changes through the year, we must nimbly shift along with it, or else we are doomed to disease.

A major point here is the danger in sudden changes. Imagine trying to balance on the wobble board when someone surprisingly jumps out of nowhere and gives a hard sudden shove. It would be almost impossible to maintain one's balance in such a situation. Contrast that with trying to balance on the board when someone slowly walks up, announces when and from which direction the push will come, and then proceeds to slowly push. It would be much easier to maintain one's balance. It's the suddenness of the change that is so dangerous. This is a point we will meet again and again. It is an important concept of ancient health. Health abhors sudden change.

What we've so far discussed is the seasonal weather patterns and how they affect our balance on the wobble board of health. But we've jumped into the weather and missed the season itself. Hippocrates makes it clear that it is not just the weather (meteorology) but the seasons themselves (astronomy) that affect us:

> If it be thought that all this belongs to meteorology, he will find out, on second thoughts, that the contribution of astronomy to medicine is not a very small one but a very great one indeed. For with the seasons men's diseases, like their digestive organs, suffer change.[8]

The world itself rejoices in the springtime. The sun returns from its long period of decline, its power returning to the world. And the world responds with growth, expansion, green, and birth. It is a time of youthfulness, laughter, and joy. The very world feels joy during this season, and we are part of this world. We may not be smiling all the time during this season, but we cannot help but sense the exuberance. The joy of this season fills us with blood. It makes us more sanguine. We become hotter and moister. Even if the weather isn't hot and moist where we live, we are still leaned by the very color of the world toward the hot and moist side of the board.

---

8   Hippocrates 1, Airs Waters Places, Ch 2.

It is likewise for each season. The summer, with the sun at its peak, blaring down upon the world, makes the world shine. But this shine is very different than the shine of springtime. It is a drying shine. The world has been hot for some time. It grows weary of the heat. Summer is a time of heat and dryness, a time when the world is active and engaged, and a time when anger erupts. It makes us bilious. Even if the weather makes the summer moist, there is still a drying effect on our lives from the very height of the sun's power and the activity it pulls forth from us.

In autumn, when the sun begins to lose its power and the world grows colder, the world itself becomes sad. Melancholy comes over us as darkness gains power in the world. The morning is darker, the angle of the light altered remarkably from the summer's blare. Black bile, cold and dry, pools in our bodies. We turn inward. We slow down. Coldness enters the world even if the weather is still hot because our internal lives, even if not our external lives, slow down. The sadness of the world makes us colder.

And in the dark of winter, when the world itself seems to have died, fear covers the earth. Will the sun ever return? Is this the end? The entire world, and even us modern people who never give it a single *conscious* thought, worry whether the world is ending. We sleep more. There is a waiting that hangs in the air. We grow moist from the stillness, stuck to the darkness of the world and of our dreams like a boot in the mud. We may not consciously sense this, but something deep inside of us feels it. We fill with phlegm, cold and moist, hoping for the return of the sun in spring.

The effect of the seasons is therefore not only the literal weather, but also the amount of sunlight, the angle of the sunlight, the changes in the trees, the changes in the wildlife. So we have two influences at work in the seasons. We have the sky and the sun and the world itself, and we have the weather, which doesn't always conform to the seasonal time, but usually follows a fairly regular pattern through the year. Both of these influences affect our balance on the wobble board of health. We need to recognize and plan for them both. The seasons themselves affect us on a very deep level, with the weather affecting us at a more superficial level.

Your Seasonal Map

It's time to get practical. We need to see how the seasonal and weather patterns affect your balance through the year. Draw a circle, marking the top 'January,' the right side 'April,' the bottom 'July,' and the left side 'October,' and divide this circle into twelve sections.

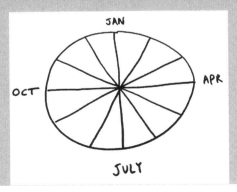

Indicate whether the weather is cold or hot in each section of the circle by placing a C for cold and an H for hot in each section of the circle. If the weather is particularly hot or cold, then underline the letter to indicate its strength, and if the weather is fairly temperate, then write the letter in lower case to indicate that it's not a strong temperature.

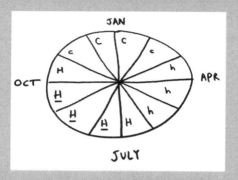

Indicate whether the weather is moist or dry in each section of the circle by placing an M for moist and a D for dry in each section of the circle. If the weather is particularly dry or moist, then underline the letter to indicate its strength, and if the weather is fairly temperate, then write the letter in lower case to indicate that it's not a strong weather pattern.

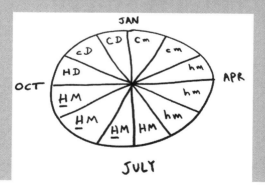

Break the circle into four quadrants by making four marks along the outside of the circle where the weather switches from hot to cold, from cold to hot, from moist to dry, and from dry to moist. Label each of the four sections: Hot/Moist, Hot/Dry, Cold/Dry, and Cold/Moist.

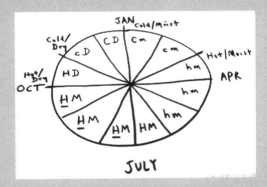

We now have a map of the weather patterns that regularly affect your life.

To understand the implications of your map, you need to look for the odd patterns. For example, let's say that where you live the weather is still hot during most of autumn. This is an odd pattern, when the season is leaning you toward the cold and dry side of the board, the weather is pushing you toward the hot side. At first glance this may seem like a nice balancing force. But the trouble is that the seasons act from a deep, inner level, while the weather acts from the outside. Odd patterns present a major challenge. In this case, the autumn season is cooling and drying you from the inside, while you simultaneously feel hot from the weather. You can easily become too cold even when feeling hot because you may lean toward the cold to cool against the hot weather and then become too cold because of the inner seasonal force that is cooling you.

For now, just note the potential problem times of the year. We will be using this Seasonal Map throughout this book.

These seasonal and weather influences affect us all, but some seem to be more affected by them than others, and some do better in some seasons and under some circumstances than others. Some people do very well in cold weather, while others do terribly. Some hate the humidity; while others get all chapped and itchy in dry weather. We each have different affinities and tolerances for certain types of weather. The reason for this is what ancient people called one's constitution.

Hippocrates says: "Of constitutions some are well or ill adapted to summer, others well or ill adapted to winter."[9] We are each born with a certain amount of heat, coldness, moisture, and dryness. Together these make our constitution. Those who were born with more heat, for example, experience disease due to heat more easily and more frequently. The hot months of the year are not the easiest of times for these people, while the cold months are usually fine. Likewise, the cold months are not the easiest of times for those born with more coldness, but the hot months are relatively easy.[10]

---

9   Hippocrates 2, Aphorisms, Book 3.

10 Hippocrates 4, Regimen 1, Ch 32.

It's easiest to imagine one's constitution as the place on which one must place one's foot on the wobble board of health. Some people, for example, are born with a lot of moisture. They have their foot glued to the moist side of the wobble board. Their entire lives are spent leaning toward the dry side of the board in order to keep from falling off into a disease of moisture.

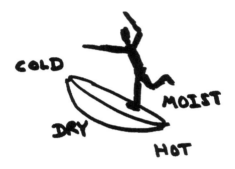

Almost all of us are born either with more heat or with more cold, and either with more moisture or with more dryness. So we each find our foot glued to one of four quadrants on the board. We are either hot and dry, hot and moist, cold and dry, or cold and moist. In the diagram below the A illustrates a person with a cold and moist constitution, with his or her foot glued in that quadrant, constantly being forced to lean his or her body toward the hot and dry side in order to stay balanced.

This picture can be further refined because most of us are not simply in the middle of a quadrant. If we have, for example, a cold and moist constitution, then usually we are either more cold than moist, or more moist than cold. Thus our foot isn't glued right in the center of a quadrant, but off to one side or the other. In the picture below, the A represents a person with a cold/moist constitution, the B represents a person with a constitution that is colder than it is moist, and the C represents a person with a constitution that is more moist than it is cold.

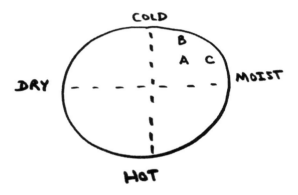

Our wobble board analogy breaks down at this point, for it's not that we either have heat or coldness, moisture or dryness. We could have lots of heat and lots of coldness, or we could have very little heat and very little coldness. Likewise, we could have lots of moisture and lots of dryness, or we could have very little moisture and very little dryness. The wobble board image is very helpful, and we will use it throughout this book, but in this regard it doesn't help us. If, for example, someone has lots of heat and lots of coldness, then he or she can easily fall off of either edge, facing a difficult time in both hot and cold environments.

It might be thought then that having just a little heat, a little coldness, a little moisture, and a little dryness would make life easy, since it would therefore be easier to keep one's balance in all directions. But although it would be easy to not get pushed off the edge by having an excess of heat, for example, there is another danger that we all face: the danger of having a deficit of heat, coldness, moisture, or dryness. We need all of them to function properly. If we run out of any of them, then disease occurs. We don't just get pushed by the forces of the world, we get pulled by them also. If we don't have enough heat, for example, then the cold can too easily pull us down into a cold disease.

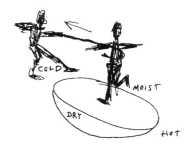

The ancients considered the ideal constitution to be that of a perfectly moderate constitution. Ideally, one has a good amount of heat, coldness, moisture, and dryness, but not too much of any. This makes it easiest to balance against excess, and makes the likelihood of deficit very low. Let's reread Galen's statement which we quoted in the *Introduction*, this time in light of the idea of the healthiest constitution:

According to our standards, the ideal body weight is midway between thin and [obese].... And likewise of the other extremes, the ideal is such that one could not call it either hirsute or bald, soft or hard, white or black, large-veined or small-veined, irascible or serene, drowsy or wakeful, sluggish or alert, voluptuous or frigid. And if the exact mean of all the extremes were in all parts of the body, this would be the best to observe as being the symmetry most suitable for all activities.[11]

The constitution that's healthiest is the constitution that most easily lends itself to maintaining balance, and that's the constitution that is moderate in all ways.

Your Constitutional Map

Let's get an image of your constitution. Draw a circle on a piece of paper, and write 'Cold' at the top, 'Moist' on the right hand side, 'Hot' at the bottom, and 'Dry' on the left hand side. Make a line connecting the moist to the dry and the hot to the cold.

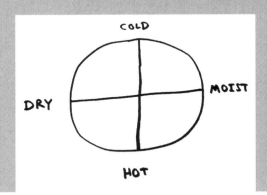

11 Hygiene. Book 1, Ch 6.

First consider whether you are more moist or dry. Moist people are usually plump ("fleshy, soft, and red"[12]), tending toward being muscular or fat. They sweat easily, and often are uncomfortable with humidity. Dry people tend to be thin ("lean and sinewy"[13]), either lean or frail. They don't sweat much, and are usually uncomfortable in dry weather, experiencing dry skin. Place a mark on the line between moist and dry indicating how much you are naturally inclined toward one of the extremes. The diagram below shows a person with a moist constitution.

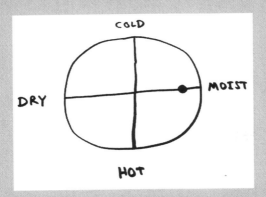

Next consider whether you are more cold or hot. Cold people often feel cold, tending to wear warm clothing. They usually are not extremely active, enjoying relaxing and calming activities. Hot people usually feel hot, wearing less or lighter clothing than other people. They are usually active and busy, tapping their feet when not actively doing something. Place a mark on the line between hot and cold indicating how much

---

12 Hippocrates 4, Regimen in Health, Ch 2.
13 Hippocrates 4, Regimen in Health, Ch 2.

you are naturally inclined toward one of the extremes. The diagram below shows a person with a hot constitution.

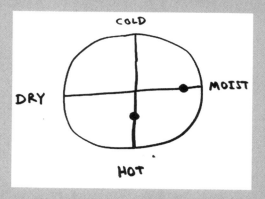

Place a mark where your two marks intersect. This mark is an image of your constitution. It shows how hot, cold, moist, and dry you are in a graphic way, making it easier to imagine how the forces of life can push and pull you around. The diagram below shows a hot and moist constitution.

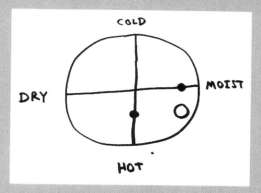

Are you hot and moist, hot and dry, cold and dry, or cold and moist? We will be using this image of your constitution throughout this book.

Let's get a clear image of how our constitutions mingle with the effects of the seasons. We are balancing on a wobble board to which our foot is glued to a greater or lesser extent toward one edge of the board, while at the same time the effects of the seasons are pushing and pulling us in various directions. We not only have to balance while the weather pushes us around, but we have to do so with our foot not centered on the board. It's a challenging task.

But that's not even the whole picture. There is one more major factor that affects our balance and over which we have no control, and that's the effect of aging. Galen makes our situation clear when he says, "... it is impossible for the body to escape the natural road to dryness, for this reason it is inevitable for us to grow old and perish...."[14] Emily Dickinson expresses it beautifully in a poem:

> Death is like the insect
> Menacing the tree,
> Competent to kill it,
> But decoyed may be.
>
> Bait it with the balsam,
> Seek it with the knife,
> Baffle, if it cost you
> Everything in life.
>
> Then, if it have burrowed
> Out of reach of skill,
> Ring the tree and leave it,—
> 'T is the vermin's will.

---

14 Hygiene, Book 6, Ch 3, p244.

The force of life puts heat and moisture into our bodies. It is the mysterious gift of life. But life itself is a great feat which can only last for so long. Over time, the heat and moisture escape, leaving us dry and cold in our old age,[15] and finally ending in death. There is no escape from aging. We are all born with more heat and with more moisture than we'll ever have again. With each passing second of our lives, we grow colder and dryer. As Hippocrates says, "... a man is warmest on the first day of his existence and coldest on his last."[16]

The easiest way to imagine the ancient idea of aging is to go back again to our wobble board. The effect of aging is to slide our foot toward the cold and the dry. Every day our foot slides just a bit more toward the cold and dry side of things, and thus we must lean a bit more toward the hot and the moist in order to stay balanced. This makes it either easier or harder for each constitution to maintain balance. If one has a hot and moist constitution, then early life is challenging because the effect of age is to lean us toward more heat and moisture. It's very hard not to fall into illness in that situation. But as one ages and the effect of age slides one toward coldness and dryness, then the board is easier to level for a hot and moist person. A person with a hot and moist constitution will likely have a tough childhood but a healthy old age. The exact opposite can be said of someone with a cold and dry constitution. The board will be easy to level in childhood, but

---

15 Hippocrates 4, Regimen 1, Ch 33.
16 Hippocrates 4, The Nature of Man, Ch 12.

as age slides one further toward the cold and dry, it will be very difficult to stay balanced.

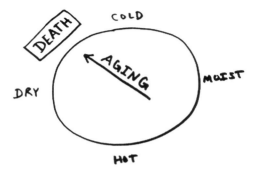

Age is slowly but relentlessly sliding the balancing foot on the wobble board toward the cold and dry edge of the board. We will eventually fall off to our deaths. But exercise is heating, and so it tilts the board slightly away from death, and food is moistening and so also turns us away from death. In this way, exercise and eating help to slow our progress toward death. We cannot stop our inevitable demise, but eating and exercising can slow the process.

In order for us to age well, we must balance the inevitable sliding toward the cold and the dry. Galen says, "... he who dries the least will live the longest."[17] Through eating and exercising, moistening and warming the body, preserving our heat and moisture, we decoy death. The ancient art of aging is to keep the body warm and moist, but, of course, not too warm and not too moist.

---

17 Hygiene, Book 6, Ch 3, p244.

It is our modern prejudice to believe that we in this advanced and progressive age live much longer and healthier lives than did the people of ancient times. We all think that we're a lot more advanced than we actually are. A statement by Galen shows us just how long they lived in ancient times:

> For there is no small difference between patients. Some being totally incapable of activity, even if they should not yet happen to be seventy years of age, and some being much stronger even though born more than eighty years before.[18]

In the ancient world, Galen was working with people in their eighties who were strong and healthy. Some of the Greeks and Romans were living as long as we do, and probably with more strength and vitality. To what can we attribute their health and longevity? Among the many possible answers to this question is their diet and exercise. Hippocrates and Galen certainly credit diet and exercise as the primary reason for health and longevity. The older one gets, the less one can tolerate too much or too little of anything, be it weather, exercise, massage, or food. So the old must take care, and the care they must take is for their diet and their exercise.

The Slippery Slope of Aging

Take a look at your Constitutional Map. How far is your foot from the cold and the dry side of the wobble board? With each passing day, your foot slides a bit closer to that side of the board until you will eventually fall to your death. It's important that you don't blindly act on old information about your constitution because your constitution is always

---

18 Hygiene. p199.

changing, always sliding toward the cold and the dry. If you are currently excessively hot and/or moist, then you will eventually become more balanced as you age. If you are currently excessively cold and/or dry, then you will become more and more imbalanced as you age. The effect of age is an important thing to consider as you plan your health practices. You should reassess your constitution on at least a yearly basis.

All that we have spoken about is important as a way to imagine the state of our health and the balance needed to maintain it. The reality is that our state of balance is always shifting. The world around us is constantly presenting us with new weather patterns that are either warmer or colder, drier or more moist. We step into an air conditioned building and get dried and cooled. We exercise and become hot. Circumstances are always changing. Life is always pushing us around, and we must be coordinated enough to keep our balance.

So far, we've discussed what happens to us and how it can imbalance us, and soon we will discuss how our diet and exercise can help to keep us balanced. But as helpful as diet and exercise can be, they can also be the cause of imbalances. Diet and exercise are powerful forces that can throw us off balance just as easily as can the seasons, our constitution, and aging. Galen says:

... some are sick all the time, not from intrinsic constitution of the body, but either on account of improper diet, or because they live an idle life, or work too hard, or error in the quality or quantity or time of their meals, or practice some injurious custom, either in the quantity of sleep, or excessive sex relations, or tormenting themselves needlessly with cares and worries. For I have known very many who are sick every year for such reasons; but we shall not say that they are poorly constituted in body, like those who, though committing none of the errors which I mentioned, are sick all the time.[19]

This quote from Galen summarizes the point quite nicely. Some of us are born into a tough situation, a constitution almost doomed to chronic imbalance and thus poor health. Others of us live in tough locations, experiencing the extremes of heat, cold, moisture, and/or dryness. Others of us are simply already quite old and will experience illness even in the best of circumstances. But most of us are actually quite well-off. We were born with reasonably healthy constitutions, we live in places that aren't ridiculously extreme, and we aren't yet so old that our health is necessarily poor. The real problem for most of us is our lifestyles.

Many of us eat terribly. And as we shall see in later sections of this book, what constitutes a healthy diet is nothing like what most of us imagine a healthy diet to be. On top of our poor dietary habits, most of us also exercise terribly. But again, as we shall see, healthy exercise is nothing like what most of us think it is. Most of us don't exercise enough, and the rest of us exercise way too much in all the wrong ways. Almost without fail, all of us think that we need way more exercise than is actually healthy for us. Most of us, even those who think they are eating and exercising in a healthy

---

19 Hygiene, Book 6, Ch 5, p248-9.

way, are not doing what Hippocrates would suggest that they do to truly be balanced and healthy. In fact, much of the common advice about healthy living is far from what Hippocrates would say.

Beyond our poor diet and exercise habits is the way in which we live our lives: Most of us simply don't have (or make) the time to take care of our health. As Galen says,

> "... to me it seems that those who through ambition or zeal have chosen some form of life so involved in affairs of business that they can have little leisure for the care of their bodies are also willing slaves to hard masters."[20]

The way we choose to live is the primary obstacle to our health.

The most important part of keeping our balance is being able to sense when we are losing it. One can't maintain balance if one doesn't even know that one is off-balance. We must learn to recognize the signs of imbalance. We also need to know how far off our balance is. Have we been only barely nudged and therefore are in need of only a slight adjustment, or are we falling face-first to the floor, requiring a large step or even a hand on the floor to keep us steady? Hippocrates says, "A wise man should consider that health is the greatest of human blessings, and learn how by his own thought to derive benefit in his illness."[21] In an effort to learn to benefit from our

---

20 Hygiene, Book 2, Ch 1, p51.
21 Hippocrates 4, Regimen of Health, Ch 9.

illnesses, we turn now to learning to recognize when and how we are imbalanced and how to rebalance ourselves.

Balancing Imbalances

"... we must endeavor to correct the disorders of health, making moister those conditions which are too dry, and making drier those which are too moist; and similarly purging the excess of those which are too warm, and restraining the excess of those which are too cool."[22] - Galen

A healthy, balanced person is comfortable at many temperatures, not often hot, cold, clammy, or chapped; is energetic, but not hyper; has a clear mind; has clear, sharp senses; sleeps soundly, but not excessively; has clear, shiny eyes; expels only a mild amount of excrement from the eyes, nose, mouth, and ears; has a regular, solid pulse; has an even breathing pattern; has a smooth, easy voice; has noticeable but not large veins that are neither hard nor soft; has a healthy complexion; doesn't suffer from skin irritations; has a big appetite, but doesn't suffer indigestion, hiccoughing, heartburn, belching, vomiting, bloatedness, or flatulence; is only occasionally thirsty; doesn't have strong desires for dry or moist foods; has smooth, easy bowel movements and isn't constipated or suffering from loose stools; is muscularly powerful, but not bulky; is trim, but not thin; has body fat, but is not fat; has a body that is limber, not stiff and not loose; sweats easily, but not profusely; and does not have achiness

---

22 Hygiene, Book 1, Ch 6.

or tension in the tissues of the body. A balanced person is the picture of health. Galen describes a balanced person in the following way:

> ... all parts of the body keep the Golden Mean, and avoid excess on either hand; excess to this are, grossness, thinness, fleshiness, leanness, fatness, hardness, softness, roughness, smoothness, all these swerve from meanness, but a man of a moderate mean temper is such an one... that if you feel his flesh, it is neither too hard nor too soft, too hot nor too cold; if you look upon his body, 'tis neither too gross nor too thin, too rough nor too smooth, neither hath it any excess or defect.[23]

An imbalanced person is someone who is missing at least one of these signs of balance. Those who are imbalanced suffer in some way in their bodies, experiencing at the very least discomfort, and often pain and debilitation. An imbalanced person is frequently uncomfortable, often feeling too hot, cold, clammy, or chapped; is either hyper or lethargic; has a dull, clouded mind or is confused; has dull senses; has disturbed sleep or sleeps excessively; has bloodshot eyes; expels very much or very little excrement from the eyes, nose, mouth, and ears; has either an irregular, fast, sharp, or soft pulse; breathes deeply, shallowly, quickly, or slowly; has a rough or muddled voice; has large, small, hard, or soft veins; has a discolored complexion that is reddish, yellowish, gray, or pale; suffers from skin irritations; has a small appetite; suffers indigestion, hiccoughing, heartburn, belching, vomiting, bloatedness, or flatulence; is either excessively thirsty or rarely thirsty; has strong desires for dry

---

23 Art. Ch 51.

or moist foods; is constipated or has loose stools; is weak or bulky; thin or fat; has a body that is stiff or loose; sweats profusely or not much at all; has achy and/or tense tissues. Galen says, "... the following are excessive, as when the body is too slender, or too fat, or too hard, or too soft, or too dry, or too moist, or too thin, or too thick...."[24] Essentially, anything that isn't reasonably balanced and even is an imbalance.

In summary, to be balanced is to feel comfortable, and to be imbalanced is to suffer from some form of discomfort. It is actually quite easy to identify if and when we are off balance. If we're uncomfortable, then we're imbalanced. But with all the different ways that we can be uncomfortable, it can seem challenging to know which direction we need to lean on the wobble board of health. We can't just realize that we have an imbalance and then correct the problem with any random remedy. We need to know which way to lean the wobble board in order to balance. If we lean to the wrong direction, then we may end up even more imbalanced.

The ancients knew that what was good for one person could be disastrous for another. Lots of exercise is needed for cold people, while to exercise much at all can be devastating for people who are too hot. So we can't make a blanket statement that exercise is a healthy thing to do. Exercise might be healthy, or it might we very unhealthy. Likewise, a diet with lots of vegetables, garlic, and olive oil, which was often prescribed by ancient doctors, works wonders for those who are too fat, for it is a very thinning diet, but for those who

---

24 Hygiene, p192.

are too thin, this kind of diet would cause major problems. There is a danger in generalizing about health. Galen dealt with this kind of generalizing almost 2,000 years ago:

> ... some men seem to be benefited and some injured by the same things. But since the bodily constitutions of many men are opposite, it is reasonable that benefit should accrue to them from opposites. ... For just as it is impossible for the cobblers to use one last for all men, so it is impossible for the physician to use one plan of life that shall be beneficial to all. Wherefore they say that for some it is healthful to exercise freely every day, but for others that nothing prevents unless they have been completely inactive; and for some bathing seems to be healthful, and for others not; and [it is the same for] drinking water and wine.... indeed I know some who, after remaining without exercise for three days, have immediately become ill; and others who never exercise, but are healthy; and some who never bathe, but are healthy; and others who, if they should not bathe, immediately have a fever....[25]

Each person is different and so needs different things and will respond in different ways to different regimens. So when we hear arguments about whether coffee, meat, milk, honey, or any other food under the sun, is good or bad for us, we should try to remember that the argument itself is faulty. Every reasonable type of food is good for some people some of the time, and bad for some people some of the time. And the same is true for all reasonable exercises too. Hot baths are great for some people, and terrible for others. Galen tells a story to illustrate this point:

---

25 Hygiene, p222-3.

... just recently two people were having an argument with each other, the one declaring that honey was healthy, the other that it was harmful, each offering as proof whatever the honey had done on an individual basis, but ignoring the fact that not everyone has the same temperament at the outset. For even if they do have just one temperament, they cannot preserve it unchanged throughout the stages of life, just as similarly they cannot preserve it through changes of season and place. ... the older of the two was by nature rather phlegmatic [cold and moist], lazy in his way of life and towards all other activities, not least the exercises in the public baths, which was why honey [which is heating and drying] was beneficial; by nature the other was bilious [hot and dry], aged thirty, and worked out a great deal with exercises every day. Understandably in this instance the honey quickly [made him excessively hot and dry], and thus was very harmful. ... indeed it is not right for them simply to talk about honey, but to add in the middle of this for which stage of life, nature, season, place and way of life it is beneficial or harmful. For example, that it is completely opposed to hot and dry things, but is most beneficial to wet and cold things, and whether this sort of person has the temperament because of age, nature, place, season or a particular lifestyle.[26]

It's ridiculous and pathetic that to this day we are still having the same useless and fruitless arguments that the Romans were having 2,000 years ago. It's time that we recognize that there is no general regimen for health because each person has a unique constitution that is affected by the unique circumstances of his or her life. We need to recognize imbalances for what they are, and identify which direction on the wobble we need to lean in order to balance our unique imbalances.

---

26 Food, p74-5.

Fortunately it's really not hard to recognize whether one is too hot, too cold, too moist, or too dry, and so it really isn't hard to figure out how to individualize things for each person. We're now going to go through each sign of imbalance and discuss their underlying causes.

Assessing Balance

If we are consistently uncomfortable in certain weather, then we are imbalanced. If we are too easily hot, then we are excessively hot, and if we are too easily cold, then we are excessively cold. Likewise, if we have trouble in humid weather, then we are too moist, and if we have trouble in dry weather, then we are too dry.

Our energy level is a major sign of our balance. If we are hyper, then we are too hot, and if we are lethargic, then we are too cold. Ideally, we are at a happy medium, energetic but not hyper, which is a sign of balance.

Our minds should be calm and quiet, not easily disturbed or confused. If our minds are wild and racy, then we are too hot. If our minds are slow and dull, then we are too cold.

Sleep should come easily and end naturally, bringing a sense of refreshment. When we have disturbed sleep, often with wild dreams, then we are too hot,[27] and if we sleep excessively and feel sleepy even after sleeping, then we are too cold.

---

27 Hygiene, p157.

There should be some excrement coming from the head, for it protects our head from the elements and keeps us from drying excessively. Having lots of excrement coming from our eyes, nose, mouth, and ears (crust in the eyes, snot, saliva, and ear wax) is a sign of excessive moisture, and having very little is a sign of excessive dryness.

Our overall balance has a large effect on our skin, and so our balance can be seen in the complexion of our skin. Our complexion should be rather neutral, ideally with a pinkish tone even for those with naturally dark skin. If the skin is reddish then we are too hot and moist; if it is orangish or yellowish, then we are too hot and dry; if the skin is dark and leaden, then we are too cold and dry; and if we are pale, then we are too cold and moist.[28]

One of the best ways for us to assess the balance of our body in general is by assessing our sweat because sweat is the way that the body in general expels waste: "... perspiration [is] indicative of the entire condition of the animal. For the warmest sensation customarily occurs in it when warm fluids prevail, and the coldest sensation when cold fluids prevail. And they appear whiter when phlegm [cold and moist fluids] prevail, and yellower when bile [hot and dry fluids] prevail...."[29] Our sweat will be thin and watery when we are too moist, and it will be thick and sticky when we are too dry. So we can notice our sweat to help us figure out our imbalances.

---

28 Hygiene, p155.
29 Hygiene, p155.

The tissues and muscles of each part of our bodies should be strong and powerful. Each tissue should look and feel supple and strong. Signs that the tissues and muscles of the body are imbalanced include them being bulky or weak, thin or fat, loose or stiff, achy or tense, hard or soft.

A body that is bulky, with excessively large muscles, is too hot and too moist. Similarly, a fat body is too cold and too moist. Excess size comes from excess moisture. A thin, wiry body is too hot and too dry. A thin, frail body is too cold and too dry. A deficit in size comes from excess dryness. In our modern world, we don't often consider large muscles and/or extreme leanness to be a sign of imbalance, but Hippocrates says that these excesses are just as imbalanced as are being fat or frail. Immoderation in any direction is an imbalance that causes disease.

In addition, the muscles, tendons, and sinews of the body should be supple, neither hard nor soft. Hardness comes from excessive tension or excessive dryness, while softness comes from excessive relaxation or excessive moisture.[30] Hard tissues must be softened into suppleness, and soft tissues must be hardened into suppleness. Similarly, looseness of a joint is caused by excessive moisture,[31] while stiffness in a joint is caused by excessive dryness.

Achy, painful tissues are inflamed with excessive heat and this can occur most easily when the body itself is too hot.[32] So

---

30 Hygiene, p193.
31 Food, p59.
32 Food, p38-9.

a painful, achy muscle or joint is a sign that the particular muscle or joint is excessively hot, and multiple muscles and joints that are painful and achy are a sign that the entire body is too hot.

Determined by the heart and the liver, our overall constitution will generally dictate the balance of the rest of our organs. Normally, the brain, lungs, stomach, and bowels will all follow the general tendency of our bodies. But this is not always the case. Sometimes one or more of the other organs will be imbalanced in its own way. Fortunately, balance is balance. In general, by balancing our constitution, we balance ourselves. If we are generally too hot and too moist, then practices that cool and dry us will help to balance us, and this balance will proceed to balance all the organs of the body. But, of course, this is also not always the case. Sometimes individual organs need individual attention. We will discuss the details of each organ in the chapter *Herbs and Remedies for Balance*. For now, we want to focus on the balance of the entire body in general.

Assessing Your Balance

It's time to assess your balance or lack thereof. Reread the previous section, this time taking note of any of your personal imbalances. Make a list of how you're imbalanced, and later you can reference this list when making a plan for how to balance yourself.

Now that we know what it's like to be imbalanced, and now that we can recognize how we are imbalanced, it is time to discuss the basics of how we might re-balance ourselves.

Hippocrates makes the process seem very simple when he says, "... counteract cold with hot, hot with cold, moist with dry and dry with moist."[33] And indeed, it is that simple. Galen helps to flesh out the details:

> And let the common object of all correction be the employment of the opposite excess, if the body has toiled too much on the previous day, by diminishing the quantity of exercise, and if too little, by increasing it; and so also if it has used too swift motions, by abating them moderately, and if too gentle, by intensifying them. And in the same way by employing gentler exercises instead of those too vigorous, and more vigorous for those too mild, and substituting the violent for the quiet, and for the violent the opposite, and comprehensively speaking, correcting all excesses by means of the opposite excess, to keep the patient healthy.[34]

We balance by balancing that which is out of balance. If we have too much of something, then we diminish it, and if we have too little of something, then we add more of it. Our primary tools for balancing are exercise, massage, bathing, eating, sleeping, and herbs.

Exercise heats, dries, and hardens the body. As we will discuss in the chapter *Exercising for Balance*, exercise can be modified so as to be anything from mildly heating to extremely heating, mildly drying to extremely drying, and mildly hardening to extremely hardening. It has both a general effect on the body, making the entire body hotter, drier, and harder, and also a specific effect on the parts of the body being exercised. For example, doing push-ups will primarily

---

33 Hippocrates 1, Ancient Medicine, Ch 8.
34 Hygiene, p192.

heat, dry, and harden the arms, and doing squats will primarily heat, dry, and harden the legs, even though both of these exercises will heat, dry, and harden the entire body to some extent.

So, if we have imbalances due to excessive cold, moisture, or softness, then exercise is a good tool for us to use. It can balance us by leaning us toward the hot and dry side of the board, and it can harden soft parts of the body. We need to be careful with exercise, since if we are already too hot, too dry, or too hard, then exercise can easily make us more imbalanced. It's important to note that exercise includes all activity in life. Just being more active in life can make us hotter, drier, and harder. It's not just a workout that counts as exercise.

Massage heats the body, and, as we will discuss in the chapter *Massaging for Balance*, massage can either moisten or dry, and either soften or harden, depending on how it is applied. As with exercise, massage has a general effect on the entire body and also a specific effect on the part of the body to which it is applied. So massaging the forearms will warm the forearms more than it will warm the rest of the body, but it will also warm the entire body to some extent.

Bathing moistens the body, and, as we will discuss in the chapter *Bathing for Balance*, if the water is warm then it will heat the body, and if it is cold then it will cool the body. Bathing has a general effect on the entire body.

Eating replenishes the body. As we will discuss in the chapter *Eating for Balance*, various foods and various ways of preparing foods can make them more or less heating, cooling, moistening, or drying. Eating has a general effect on the entire body, and can't be used to target a specific region.

Sleeping cools and moistens the body. As we will discuss in the chapter *Sleeping for Balance*, it can also soften or harden the body, depending on the surface on which we sleep. As with eating, sleeping has a general effect on the body, and can't be used to target specific regions.

Herbs can have targeted and specific effects on the body. They can heat, cool, moisten, or dry the various parts of the body, leaving the rest of the body relatively unaffected. They are potent tools for us to use to help us to stay balanced, and they are our best tools for targeting specific organs. We will discuss the details of herbs in the chapter *Herbs and Remedies for Balance*.

If we are too hot, then we can cool ourselves by modifying our exercise and massage to be less heating and by reducing the overall amount of exercise and massage that we use, and we can bathe in cool water, eat cooling foods, and get more sleep. If a particular part of the body is too hot, then we can reduce or eliminate our exercise and massage of that region, and we can use specific herbs in order to cool it.

If we are too cold, then we can warm ourselves with more exercise and massage, and we can bathe in warm water, eat warming foods, and ensure that we aren't sleeping excessively. If a particular part of the body is too cold, then we can increase our exercise and massage of that region, and we can use specific herbs to help to warm it.

If we are too moist, then we can dry ourselves with more exercise, drying massages, and shorter baths, and we can eat dryer and/or less food, and ensure that we aren't sleeping excessively. If a particular part of the body is too moist, then we can increase our exercise of the region, specifically massage the region in order to dry it, and use specific herbs to help to dry it.

If we are too dry, then we can moisten ourselves with less or even no exercise, moistening massages, and longer baths, and we can eat moistening and/or more food, and get more sleep. If a particular part of the body is too dry, then we can decrease or eliminate our exercise of the region, specifically massage the region in order to moisten it, and use specific herbs to help to moisten it.

If a part of the body is too soft, then we can harden it with vigorous exercises, hardening massage, bathing to harden the body, and sleeping on a hard surface. Exercise and massage allow us to target the soft part of the body, while bathing and sleeping can have a general hardening effect on the entire body. Likewise, if a part of the body is too hard, then we can soften it with less vigorous exercise, soft massage, bathing to soften the body, and sleeping on a soft surface. Exercise and massage allow us to target the hard part of the body, while bathing and sleeping can have a general softening effect on the entire body.

These tools that we have at our disposal (exercise, massage, bathing, eating, sleeping, and herbs) are extremely useful and very powerful. They are our only way of staying balanced and healthy. They're how we can adjust ourselves on the wobble board of health. But as useful as they can be, they can also be destructive. They can throw us off balance just as easily as they can balance us. It is all in how they are applied. For example, excessive or misapplied exercise can ruin our balance very quickly. We all know how excessive eating can make us very unhealthy, and imagine how quickly we'd get into trouble if we stopped eating entirely.

The basic guideline for how to make use of our tools for health is to use them all moderately. We all need some amount of exercise, but never to fatigue. Massage is usually very helpful for balancing, but it should never drain our energy or leave our tissues too hard or too soft. Bathing should never leave us pruned, and it should never make us feel excessively hot or leave us chilled. Eating should never cause us indigestion. And sleeping should always restore us, not leave us fatigued.

Moderation is a very obvious strategy. We should do a moderate amount of moderate exercise each and every day. We should eat a moderate amount of moderate foods each and every day. When we eat something hot, we should have something cold to balance it out. We should take tepid baths that are not too long and not too short, and not too cold and not too hot. We should massage daily, but not too much or too little, and not too soft or too hard. All things in moderation. That's the name of the game for balancing health.

It seems so easy, but moderation is a challenge. Many of us are imbalanced not from the weather or from our constitutions, but from immoderate use of eating and exercising. Galen says, "The habit of mind is impaired by faulty customs in food and drink and exercise and sights and sounds and music."[35] So there are two types of imbalances: those caused by things that we cannot control, such as the season, the weather, our constitution, and aging, and those caused by things which we can control, namely exercise, massage, bathing, eating, sleeping, and herbs. It is truly a shame to be imbalanced because of something that we can control. For example, to be too dry from excessive exercise is to be imbalanced from something that should help to make us balanced, not imbalanced. Galen says, "I say when the body needs rest, idleness is better than exercise, for that helps nature when the other weakens it."[36] And Hippocrates says,

... diseases due to repletion are cured by evacuation, and those caused by evacuation are cured by repletion; those due to exercise are cured by rest, and those due to idleness are cured by exercise.... relax what is tense and make tense what is relaxed.[37]

If we use any of our tools immoderately, then it will lead to imbalance. It's important to understand that we must deal with

---

35 Hygiene, Book 1, Ch 8.
36 Art. Ch 85.
37 Hippocrates 4, The Nature of Man, Ch 9.

this problem at the level of the problem. Poor eating habits, for example, must be addressed with diet, not with exercise. This seems so obvious, but it is a common mistake. Many people try to deal with excessive exercise by using massage to soften their excessively hard muscles. This kind of strategy can go on for years, ruining the body and its balance in the process. Many people overeat and then try to use excessive exercise to balance it out. But we must address the problem at its source instead.

A similar example happens when we are too active in our lives or when we exercise too much, causing ourselves to dry out. We become too dry and really need moisture, and food is our primary source of moisture. But eating excessive amounts of food in the hope of balancing out the excess dryness due to excessive activity will not lead to balance. The excess food cannot be properly processed by our bodies and will end up as clumps of fatty tissue in our bodies and large pools of waste material. In this situation we would want to ensure that we are getting adequate amounts of food and that the food is very moistening, but we would not want to fight excess with excess. The obvious answer is to reduce our activity level.

Similarly, if we are too dry because of excessively long exercise sessions, and we try to balance it with longer baths, then we may have some amount of success, but the root cause is not being addressed. The real problem is that we are exercising for excessively long periods of time, and we need to change this to truly balance ourselves. Likewise, if we are too dry because we are not moistening ourselves appropriately with baths and massage, and we try to balance ourselves by decreasing the length of our exercise sessions, then we again may partially balance ourselves, but the real problem is that we need to moisten ourselves more appropriately, not to stop exercising.

The bottom line is that immoderate use of our balancing tools can imbalance us, and this is a common problem that is affecting most of us. We need to recognize when our health regimen is actually making us less healthy.

Excessive exercise can dry the head, making it feel heavy and stiff.[38] It can also make one sleepy, having heavy eyelids and many yawns even after sleeping.[39] Another sign is a poor response to exercise, with trembling of the body and chills when exercising.[40] If we are imbalanced from excessive exercise, then our solution is simple: exercise less. We should reduce our exercise by at least half, eat more food, oil and massage ourselves, take warm baths, and just take it easy. Hippocrates makes it clear: "These patients ought to take their baths warm, to sleep on a soft bed, to get drunk once or twice, but not to excess, to have sexual intercourse after a moderate indulgence in wine, and to slack off their exercises, except walking."[41]

Eating, like exercise, can be imbalancing if used inappropriately. The main thing that excessive food does is

---

38 Hippocrates 4, Regimen, Book 3, Ch 83.
39 Hippocrates 4, Regimen, Book 3, Ch 84.
40 Hippocrates 4, Regimen, Book 3, Ch 84.
41 Hippocrates 4, Regimen, Book 3, Ch 85.

that it causes excessive waste material in the body. There is simply more junk left over from the food than our bodies can expel, and this excessive waste material builds up and causes problems. The earliest and most obvious signs of excess food are digestive problems because the body attempts to deal with the problem right there where it starts, in the digestive tract. These signs include constipation, diarrhea, flatulence, belching, and heartburn.[42]

If the excess of food continues, creating more and more waste material, then it begins to spill over into the rest of the body. It can fill out heads, making us sleepy with heavy eyelids, especially after eating and sleeping.[43] It can fill our sinuses with junk, especially after eating and sleeping, blocking our nostrils, and making our forehead itchy.[44] It can also make our head feel heavy,[45] and give us distressing sleep.[46] It can decrease our appetite for food and drink, and give us a faded complexion.[47] The excess waste can also create a situation in which the entire body is overwhelmed by the waste material, giving us an achy feeling as if we had exercised too much,[48] making us think that we should rest and eat, when the opposite is actually the case.

---

42 Hippocrates 4, Regimen, Book 3, Ch 73-77.
43 Hippocrates 4, Regimen, Book 3, Ch 71.
44 Hippocrates 4, Regimen, Book 3, Ch 70.
45 Hippocrates 4, Regimen, Book 3, Ch 73.
46 Hippocrates 4, Regimen, Book 3, Ch 73.
47 Hippocrates 4, Regimen, Book 3, Ch 70.
48 Hippocrates 4, Regimen, Book 3, Ch 72.

Exercise is one of the best ways to expel waste material, and so often the signs of excessive food can be blamed on insufficient exercise. If one isn't exercising enough, then waste material can easily become excessive. Without adequate exercise, we are almost doomed to experiencing excess waste in our bodies, having chronic digestive troubles, being tired and sleepy, having a stuffy nose, and achiness in our bodies. But we must be careful here, because exercise also creates its own waste material as it burns the fuel stored in the body. Exercise helps expel waste, but it can't help us if we've already overloaded the body with excessive food. So we can't use excessive exercise to balance excessive food. This is a prime example of when we need to be careful to distinguish the cause of our imbalance. If we are imbalanced because we aren't exercising, then we need exercise, and if we're imbalanced because we eat too much, then we need to eat less.

In all situations when excess food has caused an imbalance, which are dangerous periods when the body has already been pushed too far, we must reduce our exercise in order to prevent even more waste from accumulating. Our exercise must be gentle and primarily used for the purpose of expelling the excess waste. Warm baths and walking both help to expel the waste material and bring us back to balance.[49] Once the excess food waste has been resolved, we are safe to increase our exercise to a healthy, balanced level. Obviously, we must decrease the quantity of our food intake in this situation.

---

49 Hippocrates 4, Regimen, Book 3, Ch 70, 72.

If we exercise excessively, then we'll end up too hot and dry, and if we don't exercise enough, then we'll end up cold and moist. Immoderate exercising and immoderate eating both lead to imbalance. Almost all readers will fall into one of four categories: those who exercise too much and eat too much and so become excessively large and muscular, those who exercise too much and don't eat enough and so become excessively lean, those who don't exercise enough and don't eat enough and so become frail, and those who don't exercise enough and eat too much and so become fat. The diagram below illustrates the four common excesses due to immoderate exercising and eating. Very few of us are actually exercising and eating moderately, and therefore very few of us are well-balanced.

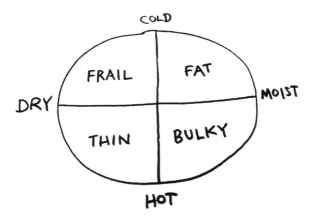

We must endeavor to catch ourselves behaving immoderately, and to correct the imbalances in our regimens. Galen gives us great advice:

... [weather] to a body of the best constitution, a moderate quantity of both meat and drink, sleeping and [activity], motion and rest, etc, is convenient, but when the air is distempered, you must vary the rest accordingly, that so the body may neither shame for cold, nor sweat for heat; as for motion, when your body begins to be weary, leave off exercise; the quantity of good is known by the perfectness of the digestions, and the waste voided ought to be according to the quantity of the food taken in; for a good nature, appetites no more than it concocts; and the contrary shows a failing in nature; also nature when it is strong is bale to set bounds to sleep, and when the body needs no more, the man wakes, there is no failing in the excrements, of urine, dung, etc, and if you consider this but well, you may easily see such a man is not easily moved by affections of the mind: anger, sadness, fury, fear, envy, etc, for these alter the body from its natural state.[50]

The basic plan is very simple: everything in moderation. Exercise, massage, bathe, eat, and sleep, all in moderation. And when that basic plan cannot keep us balanced, due to things that we cannot control, such as our constitution, the seasons, or our age, then we slightly modify our regimen in order to restore and maintain our balance. This is the basic plan for health. All we must do is follow a moderate daily regimen for health, and make small adjustments as the seasons change.

As simple as this basic plan sounds, we need to remember that health abhors sudden change. We can't make large, sudden changes in our regimen and expect good results. We need to anticipate the changes in the weather and the

---

50 Art. Ch 85.

seasons, and plan accordingly, making small changes to our regimen in preparation for the changes in circumstances. Hippocrates says:

> ... eating alone will not keep a man well; he must also take exercise. For food and exercise, while possessing opposite qualities, yet work together to produce health. For it is the nature of exercise to use up material, but of food and drink to make good deficiencies. And it is necessary, as it appears, to discern the power of the various exercises, both natural exercises and artificial, to know which of them tends to increase flesh and which to lessen it; and not only this, but also to proportion exercise to bulk of food, to the constitution of the patient, to the age of the individual, to the season of the year, to the changes of the winds, to the situation of the region in which the patient resides, and to the constitution of the year. A man must observe the risings and setting of stars, that he may know how to watch for change and excess in food, drink, wind and the whole universe, from which diseases exist among men.[51]

The next six chapters of this book will cover the details of exercise, massage, bathing, eating, sleeping, and herbs. The idea is to understand how each of these tools can be used to specifically keep us in balance and to prevent them from throwing us off balance, and how we can gradually adjust them through the changing seasons of the year to balance ourselves against the imbalancing forces of life.

---

51 Hippocrates 4, Regimen 1, Ch 2.

Exercising for Balance

*"For above all it is necessary to preserve our bodily
warmth within the limits of health. And it is preserved
by moderate exercise.... But excessive activity...
[makes] the animal [too hot and dry], and deficient
activity makes him too [too cold and moist]..."[52] - Galen*

Living our lives is exercise. Getting out of bed, walking
around, cleaning the house, carrying groceries, doing yard
work. Our daily life is exercise. But to Hippocrates, even more
than this was exercise. Seeing things, hearing things, even
thinking things, was a form of exercise. Feeling emotions was
part of exercise.[53] Even if one is bedridden, one is still
exercising if one is visited by friends, seeing people, hearing
stories, and experiencing emotions. Even if one sits all day at
a desk, one is still exercising if one is thinking hard, or if one
is worried or anxious all day about something.

All these forms of exercise have one major thing in common:
they all generate heat. Living one's life generates heat. It
keeps the internal fire alive. It fans the flame of life. Lying in
bed all day, not engaging with the world, not seeing, doing, or
thinking of much, is what leads to the dwindling of the spark
of life. The primary purpose of exercise is to keep that spark

---

52 Hygiene, Book 1, Ch 8.
53 Hippocrates 4, Regimen 2, Ch 61.

alive. We must exercise daily, even if only in the form of living our lives, in order to fan the flame of life. In this chapter we're going to discuss the use of exercise as a tool to help us to keep our balance, that is, to take exercise in the form of a workout, as an act we perform to balance our health.

We all fall into one of two categories: those who tend toward too much exercise, and those who tend toward too little. Those who tend to do too much exercise desperately need the following advice from both Hippocrates and Galen:

> Perhaps it would be claimed that athletes achieve some of the physical blessings. Will they claim the most important blessing: health? You will find no one in a more treacherous physical condition, if we are to believe Hippocrates, who said that the extreme good health for which they strive is treacherous. ... For [Hippocrates] proposed for a program in health: "Work, food, drink, sleep, love, and all in moderation." But athletes overexert every day at their exercises, and they force-feed themselves, frequently extending their meals until midnight.

> Thus too, their sleep is immoderate. When normal people have ended their work and are hungry, the athletes are just getting up from their naps. In fact, their lives are just like those of pigs, except that pigs do not overexert nor force-feed themselves.

> ... the extreme conditioning of athletes is treacherous... for there is no room for improvement and it cannot remain constant, and so the only way that remains is downhill.

> But perhaps [athletes] will claim... that they have strength, indeed, that they are the strongest of men. But, in the name of the gods, what kind of strength is this, and good for what?

Can they do agricultural work such as digging or harvesting or plowing? But perhaps their strength is good for warfare? Euripides will tell us, for he said: "Do men fight battles with [the discus] in their hands?" Are they strong in the face of cold and heat? Are they rivals of Hercules so that they too, summer or winter, sleep under the heavens? In all these respects they are weaker than newborn babies.[54]

Those who tend toward too little exercise can take comfort that there is no reason that exercise need be a major burden in life. No one needs to train like an athlete to be healthy.

The main reason that we exercise is to preserve our bodily warmth within the limits of a healthy balance. Being active during the day is exercise, and it warms us. So we take exercise in the form of a workout primarily to overcome the effects of a cold constitution, cold weather, or lack of activity in our lives. But exercise does more for us than just warm us. It also expels waste material from our bodies, which is no small consequence. Waste material builds up in our bodies and can easily cause us severe imbalances if it is not expelled readily. Exercise is a powerful help in this process. In addition, exercise strengthens our bodies, keeping us from getting injured in our daily lives. In essence, exercise heats us and dries us, cleanses us of waste, and strengthens us.

In order to best understand the benefits of exercise, we should first focus on what happens when we don't exercise enough. Insufficient exercise causes a lack of warmth which leaves us too cold, too moist, too weak, and too full of waste.

---

54 Galen quoted by Miller. *Arete*. Los Angeles: University of California Press: 1991. P174-6.

So lack of exercise makes us more likely to get injured, excessively moist, full of waste, and excessively cold.

One might argue that all any of us need to do for exercise is to walk in order to maintain our warmth and expel waste, so that walking is the only exercise that any of us ever need. But that would be to ignore one very important reason that we exercise: we exercise to keep our bodies strong enough to not get injured by our daily lives. Some of us lead more strenuous lives than others, but we all need some amount of strength or else our tissues will get injured too easily from our day-to-day lives. For example, we need to be strong enough to carry groceries up the stairs. If one is an athlete, then one must be strong enough to perform one's sport and not get hurt. We cannot only do gentle exercise and expect to be strong enough to not break down by the nature of life. We need both gentle and vigorous exercises if we are to be healthy. Vigorous exercise makes us stronger so that we can tolerate life. Of course, we don't need to be extremely strong to be healthy, but we do need a reasonable level of strength, and this can only be developed by vigorous exercise. We need just enough vigorous exercise to keep us strong enough and powerful enough that our daily lives don't cause us injury.

In a similar way, we need to have enough endurance in order to not end up exhausted from our daily lives. So we can't only do gentle exercise and expect to be enduring enough to not break down by the nature of life. We need swift exercises that challenge our endurance if we are to be healthy. The swift exercises make us more enduring so that we can tolerate life.

Of course, we don't need to be extremely enduring to be healthy, but we do need a reasonable level of endurance, and this can only be developed by swift exercises. We need just enough vigorous and swift exercises to keep us strong and enduring enough that our daily lives won't cause us to be overwhelmed.

Galen provides a wonderful definition of exercise: "if anyone is compelled by any movement to breathe more or less faster, that movement becomes exercise for him."[55] So any movement that causes a change in one's breathing is exercise. If it makes us breathe harder than usual, such as when running, then it is challenging enough to be considered swift exercise. And if it makes us breathe slower, holding our breath or grunting in order to complete the exercise, such as when pushing against a heavy weight, then it is vigorous enough to strengthen us. The great thing about this definition of exercise is that it individualizes the notion of exercise. If the weight is heavy enough to make one slightly grunt while doing it, then it is a heavy enough weight to be considered vigorous exercise. If one is walking fast enough or running fast enough to notice that one's breathing is faster than when going about one's daily activities, then it's fast enough to be considered swift exercise. Anything that meets this requirement is enough to do what we need exercise to do. It will tone the body's tissues, help expel waste, and warm and dry the body.

A very strong man might pick up a 100# barrel without a change in his breathing, while an average man would have to

---

55 Hygiene, p53-4.

hold his breath in order to pick it up. For the strong man, lifting 100# is not exercise, but for the average man it is. Likewise, a trained athlete can run a ten-minute mile without even increasing his breathing rate, while an untrained couch-potato would be panting to run such a pace. What is considered exercise is thus different for different people.

Galen's simple definition of exercise helps us to easily identify what is enough exercise without needing any objective measurements, timing devices, scales, etc. It is an utterly subjective measurement, something that is determined by quality, not quantity. By using his definition of exercise, we learn to sense what is enough, instead of needing to be told what is enough. From this definition of exercise, we can now easily tell whether an exercise is vigorous enough to strengthen us or swift enough to make us more enduring. If we have to slightly hold our breath or grunt when we perform the exercise, then it is vigorous enough to make us stronger. And if we have to breathe harder and faster than normal, then it is fast enough to make us more enduring.

We need to remember that we are exercising for health - to keep ourselves balanced - not for fitness, sport performance, pleasure, to burn calories, or to look better in the mirror. Of course, the exercise we take for health reasons may very well make us look better, improve our performance, and make us feel good, but that is not the reason that we do it. We do it to balance on the wobble board. Exercising for health is thus a safe way to exercise. For if we get lost in the goal of trying to look better in the mirror or trying to shave a few more seconds off our mile run, then we can easily exercise excessively, overheating and over-drying the body, and leading us into disease and injury. But because we are only interested in balancing ourselves, there is never a reason to come even close to hurting ourselves with exercise.

Since exercise keeps our bodies functioning well, we should take it daily. Daily exercise is healthy exercise. Exercising less frequently than daily, three times per week for example, allows one to do more in each workout and requires more rest. Since we know that we'll get lots of rest after our three-times-per-week workout, it's all too easy to exercise too much and end up injured by infrequent exercise. In addition, it keeps us from fanning the flame of life on a daily basis, and from daily toning our organs and tissues. Less frequent exercise is called "training," and it's what athletes need, not what average people need. Galen makes this clear:

> ... it is necessary for athletes, in order that they may prepare themselves for their labors in competitions, to practice immoderately sometimes all day at their objective exercise, which they call training. But for those exercising for the sake of health alone, it is not necessary nor at all useful to be led into excessive labor, so that there is no fear of incurring fatigue.[56]

Exercise is good, but too much of it can be very harmful. Hippocrates, Galen, and Plato all warn against the pursuit of extreme athletic fitness as the following quotes make clear.

---

56 Hygiene, p101.

Hippocrates says: "The athletic state is not natural; better the healthy condition."[57] And Galen says:

> The extreme of this athletic state, which is [the athlete's] ultimate aim, actually endangers their health.[58]

> Health consists in a certain kind of balance; [athletic training] creates imbalance, by increasing the amount and density of the flesh, and producing a quantity of blood which is, in simple terms, extremely sticky. For its aim is to increase not only strength, but also the bulk and weight, of the body, as these too assist in the worsening of one's antagonist. It is therefore not a difficult conclusion to draw that the practice is in this way detrimental to the performance of natural functions, as well as leading to other kinds of danger.[59]

Plato says:

> ... this redundant type of care of the body [athletic training], which goes beyond the dictates of gymnastics, would appear to be the worst of all. It causes problems to the management of a household, to military actions, and to the conduct of civic offices. The biggest problem, though, is that it prevents any kind of learning, contemplation, or study; for there is the fear that some kind of strain or swimming in the head may arise from the practice of philosophy; so that it is an absolute hindrance in any context where philosophical virtue is pursued and held in esteem. For it gives one the impression of being in a constant state of fatigue and bodily pain.[60]

---

57 Hippocrates quoted by Galen in Selected. P87.
58 Selected. P87.
59 Selected. P87-8.
60 Plato quoted by Galen in Selected.

The sort of exercise needed to excel in athletics requires a very strict regimen to balance its effects. Most people can't handle this balance and will get disease.[61] For those seeking health, the athletic style of training is not the answer. Simple, mildly challenging, daily exercise is the key.

The results of taking daily exercise are wonderful. First of all, the health effects of expelling waste, warming the body, mobilizing the joints and soft tissues, practicing good movement patterns, and 'blowing-off steam' and excess energy, are all wonderful daily events. Injuries and overtraining become less likely because one knows that one will have to do it again the next day. Exercise time is reduced each day, so that it doesn't take forever to get through a workout. Daily exercise also significantly reduces exercise soreness because it forces one to do less in any given workout and simultaneously works the range of motion and pumps the tissues that would otherwise be sore in order to resolve soreness very rapidly and prevent it from ever developing in the first place.

For health purposes, daily exercise is the way. This chapter's emphasis is not on whether we should exercise or not, because we should exercise daily if health is our concern. What this chapter is about is how we can modify our workouts so that they help to keep us balanced, and so that they don't end up throwing us off balance.

The wonderful benefits of exercise can also be detriments. Exercise can overheat us, over-dry us, create excessive

_____
61 Hippocrates 4, Aphorisms, Ch 1.

waste, and cause us injury. The prevention of these various dangers is the most important part of learning to exercise well. Galen says: "The art of exercise is no small part of [staying healthy], and avoiding fatigue is no small part of the art of exercise."[62] This is a very important point: preventing fatigue and injuries is one of the keys to exercising well.

There are five main ways that exercise can harm us. The first we have already discussed, and that is that is can overheat and overdry us. We must always be on guard to ensure that exercise is only heating and drying us enough to help us to stay balanced, and no more. But there are a number of other ways that exercise can hurt us, and we need to address each in turn. Hippocrates[63] and Galen[64] tell us about injury and fatigue, and they tell us how to prevent it. The following discussion of fatigue draws heavily from their works.

Exercise is challenging. It necessitates that we use force, and too much force can cause injury. There are three levels of excessive force. The first occurs when we use a mild amount of excessive force. This causes our tissues, our muscles, tendons, ligaments, and joints, to tighten in response to the excessive force placed upon them. Galen called this Tension Fatigue. The body becomes tight in response to excessive force. This restricts our ability to move, and is often the first step toward severe injuries and chronic pain.

---

62 Hygiene, p143.
63 Hippocrates 4, Regimen 2, Ch 66.
64 Hygiene, Book 3, Ch 5-7.

There are two main ways to end up with Tension Fatigue. When a person is deconditioned, simply too weak for daily life, then that person can end up with Tension Fatigue because daily life can overload a weak body. The other way to get Tension Fatigue is by using too vigorous of exercises in one's workout. It's important to keep the force required to complete one's workout within reasonable and safe limits. We need to always remember that if the resistance we are working against requires us to mildly grunt or hold our breath in order to complete the exercise, then it is enough to strengthen us. We don't need to blindly add resistance ad nauseum.

A step beyond Tension Fatigue is tendinitis, when the tissues become severely inflamed and irritated from excessive force. This can happen from the use of moderately excessive force, or from Tension Fatigue being ignored until it worsens. The step beyond tendinitis is rupture, when a tissue of the body tears and is severely damaged, which occurs from either severely excessive force or from the continued ignoring of the warnings of the body. Tension Fatigue will continue to develop into worse conditions unless properly managed.

Galen tells us how to manage Tension Fatigue. The affected regions will be inflexible. What is needed is relaxation of the tissues to help them to soften from hardness to balance. Most importantly, one must reduce the force required from exercise and perhaps take a complete rest from certain exercises. Temperate baths with a long stay in warm water can help to relax the affected areas. A little bit of gentle massage with oil can help a lot, but it's important to never use hard pressure on parts of the body that are already hardened. The tension will only relax in response to gentle massage. Of course, preventing Tension Fatigue is best. Besides ensuring that we don't use excessive force when we exercise, the best way to prevent Tension Fatigue is by properly warming up for exercise.

Tension Fatigue can happen to anyone, not only the relatively weak. For example, a man who can only lift 50# overhead will get Tension Fatigue if he tries to lift 55# overhead, and so will a man who can lift 100# who tries to lift 105#. A person's strength doesn't matter if they are trying to do more than they can tolerate. But there is a big difference between these two men. The stronger man, who can lift 100#, is much less likely to be overloaded by his daily life than is the weaker man. One of the major reasons to exercise is to become reasonably strong, to have enough strength that reasonable daily activities do not overwhelm us, so that we do not get Tension Fatigue or other injuries from our daily lives.

Another major problem that can occur from exercise is caused by the waste products formed when we exercise. The ancients imagined that the flesh of the body was melted during exercise. That's a great way to imagine it, and it is a fairly accurate picture of what is mechanically occurring. When we exercise, our muscles burn our fat and glycogen that is stored in the body. When these are broken down for fuel, there is waste material left over. The waste material pools in the body and it must be removed. If the body is unable to adequately remove the waste material, then it can sit in our muscles for days and cause a very unpleasant burning sensation when we move. Galen called this Ulcerous Fatigue.

Ulcerous Fatigue can be caused by excessive amounts of any type of exercise, but it is more commonly caused by swift exercises such as running. It gives us a distressing sensation when we move, often at the skin level. Galen recommends preventing this type of fatigue by never doing an excessive amount of exercise, and by always assisting the body in removing the waste after exercise. There are three things we can do to assist the body to remove the waste, all of them involving an adequate cool-down after exercise. If we stop suddenly after exercise then there is little way for the body to purge the waste away. By taking the time to do a cool-down after exercise, we help the body to remove the waste. Going for a walk is an excellent way to help the body to purge waste material. The gentle movement of walking keeps the body moving, allowing it to more easily remove the waste without adding significant stress to the body. Finishing a workout with massage and stretching, both of which help to squeeze the tissues of the body so that the waste material can be more easily moved through the body, are the other two keys to preventing Ulcerous Fatigue. Proper massage and stretching after a workout is called apotherapy by Galen, and was one of the most highly recommended components of a healthy exercise routine. If we end each workout by walking, massaging, and stretching, then the odds of being overloaded by waste material are small.

If Ulcerous Fatigue does occur, then Galen has the following suggestions to help in its recovery. We should take gentle massage with oil, and do apotherapeutic exercises, which are moderate, gentle movements done slowly with many pauses. This helps to expel the waste material from the body. We should take a little less food than normal, and have it be a little bit more moist, especially to prevent it from becoming Dry Fatigue, which we'll discuss below. Starchy foods are known to hinder the expelling of excrement, and so should be avoided during the recovery from Ulcerous Fatigue.

The final type of fatigue that exercise can cause is very similar to Ulcerous Fatigue in cause, but very different in nature. It was called Dry Fatigue by Galen. This occurs when one exercises for an excessively long period so as to cause such a loss of moisture that it cannot be adequately replenished. The body shrinks and dries up. This should be prevented by never exercising for too long. But when it does occur, one must bathe, preferably in cold water, and eat lots of moist foods in order to replenish the loss of moisture.

Even though we should take precautions against excessive exercise so that in an ideal situation we are never fatigued or injured, the nature of life will cause us to be at least sometimes fatigued by exercise. To this, Hippocrates has great advice for us: "Such as are fatigued after their running ought to wrestle; such as are fatigued by wrestling ought to run. For by taking exercise in this way they will warm, brace and refresh best the part of the body suffering from fatigue."[65]

---

65 Hippocrates 4, Regimen of Health, Ch 7.

The basic idea is that when we are fatigued by one form of exercise, we should change to another form. If running is causing us problems, then we should try weightlifting, and if weightlifting is causing us problems, then we should switch to running.

Tension Fatigue occurs from too much quality of work, that is, from too much force. Ulcerous and Dry Fatigue occur from too much quantity of work, when we either create too much waste material from too much work or we use up too much of our reserves from too much work. The common denominator is excess work. To prevent these problems, we must err on the side of doing less: "... for those exercising for the sake of health alone, it is not necessary nor at all useful to be led into excessive labor, so that there is no fear of incurring fatigue."[66] There is a balance to be struck here. We need to do enough to adequately strengthen, expel waste, warm, and dry the body, but not so much so as to cause fatigue: "Clearly the exerciser must not be too ambitious, so that he is still eager to exercise when his strength is already weary, nor lazy so as to give up while still able to work."[67]

So, then, how far should we push ourselves? Are we to continue to the finish line without breaking a sweat? Are we to push it to the point of failure, almost vomiting to reach our goals? The answer is simple: exercise is to be done to the start of discomfort. We rest immediately upon discomfort,[68] fatigue, or a breakdown in form. For health purposes, we

66 Hygiene, p102.
67 Hygiene, p76.
68 Hippocrates 4, Aphorisms, Book 2, Ch 48.

need to learn to mildly challenge ourselves at prescribed amounts of work. For example, if running 400m would be a balancing exercise for us to do, then we need to learn to run 400m at a mildly challenging pace. That is, a pace that makes us breathe hard, sweat, and not want to continue at that pace after we've finished the run. It's not a pace that we could sustain for another 400m, and it's not a pace that knocks us on the ground once we've finished. It's a slightly uncomfortable pace. Similarly, for lifting weights, if doing a set of five repetitions of overhead presses would be balancing for us, then we want to use a weight that will be mildly challenging for us to accomplish five repetitions. By the fourth or fifth repetition of the set, we should be slightly grunting, but not scared that we're going to drop the weight, and certainly not so unchallenged that we could keep going for another five repetitions. It takes time to learn how to mildly challenge oneself. But if we always start by erring on the side of doing too little, and then build from there, it is a fairly simple process. We jog around the track for 400m the first time, and then go a little faster and a little faster each time until it becomes mildly challenging. We do a set of five repetitions with a weight that could easily be done for ten repetitions, and build from there, adding a small amount of weight each time.[69]

Whether one currently exercises too much or too little, the solution is to start exercising moderately. Those who haven't exercised enough will need to start with a little bit of exercise and slowly work toward doing more, and those who have exercised too much will also need to start with a little bit of

---

69 Hygiene, p93-95.

exercise to allow their bodies to recover from the excess. So all readers should start with a gentle exercise regimen and then slowly build into a moderate regimen.

Basic Workout

A workout should always consist of three main phases: 1) the warm-up, 2) the workout proper, and 3) the cool-down (which the ancients called apotherapy). We will discuss each phase in detail.

Warm-Up: Preparatory Massage and Movements

Health abhors sudden change, and so going from cold to hot too quickly, which is what happens when we exercise vigorously without adequately warming-up, is a very common way to injure the body. The same person doing the exact same workout could achieve healthy, balancing effects, or could get serious injuries and imbalances, all depending on whether he or she prepares the body properly for the endeavor or not. A warm-up prepares the tissues of the body by warming them and by preparing them for the rigors of exercise. By heating the body, the warm-up dilates the pores and helps to expel waste, preventing Ulcerous Fatigue, and by preparing the body for vigorous exercise it helps to prevent Tension Fatigue.

The most important part of a warm-up is that each part of the body is flushed and ready for action. Most people have certain parts of the body that are colder than others and which require a more thorough warm-up. Each person needs to recognize his or her cold regions, which are often cold to the touch and therefore easily identifiable. These parts of the body need to be emphasized during the warm-up.

There are three components to a warm-up. The first is preparatory massage. We massage the entire body to prepare it for exercise. The purpose of preparatory massage is to warm the entire body.

A few strokes with the hands is all that is necessary to prepare each part of the body.[70] We start with a gentle stroke and build to a firm stroke, taking perhaps five strokes to build the pressure. The firm pressure helps to ready the tissues for the vigorous work to come, preventing injuries.[71]

Preparatory Massage

The entire preparatory massage can be done in standing. The following sequence works well.

Perform each of these massage strokes about five times, starting with a gentle pressure and building to a firm but comfortable pressure.

Head and Neck Massage. With both hands, stroke from your forehead over your head and down the back of your neck, finishing by sliding your hands forward to rub the sides of your neck.

---

70 Hygiene, p56.
71 Hygiene, p73.

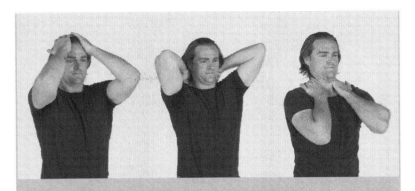

Shoulder Blade Massage. With your left hand, reach as far down and back along your right shoulder blade and mid-back muscles as you can, and then stroke upward and over the upper part of your right shoulder.

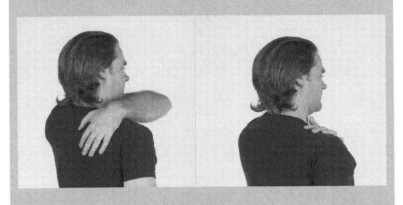

Lat and Pec Massage. With your left hand, reach as far across your body to the right side of your lower back as you can, and then stroke upward to your right armpit and then forward across your chest.

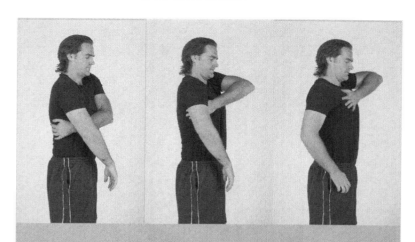

Arm Massage. With your left hand, reach as far behind your right shoulder as you can, and then stroke downward along the back of your right arm, over your shoulder, tricep, and back of the forearm, then return with a stroke that wraps to the front of your right forearm and up across your bicep, and then wraps over your shoulder, preparing for another downward stroke.

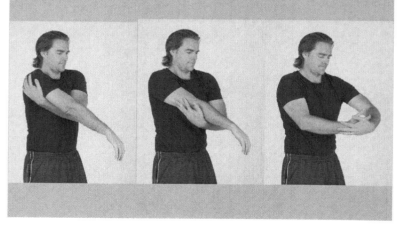

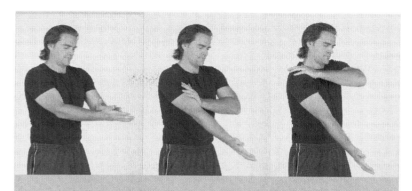

Hand Massage. With your left hand, stroke from your right wrist down the length of the palm toward each finger.

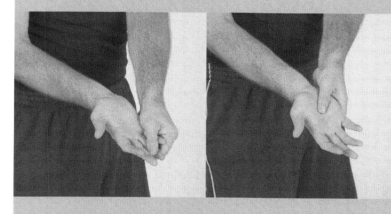

Repeat the massage of the shoulder blade, lat and pec, arm, and hand on the left side.

Abdominal Massage. With both hands, stroke from the bottom of the front of your ribs downward to the front of your pelvis.

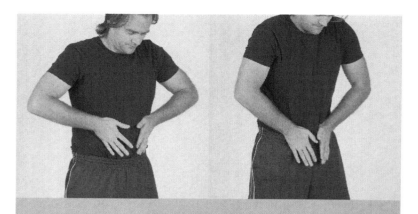

Low Back and Pelvic Massage. With each hand, stroke from as high as each hand can reach on your low back downward over your low back muscles and ending at your tailbone.

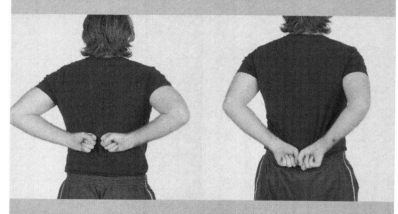

Front of the Thigh Massage. With each hand, stroke from the upper and outer part of your thighs downward and inward to the inside of your knees, and then return with a stroke upward along your inner thigh that crosses back to the outer part of the upper thigh near the top of your thighs.

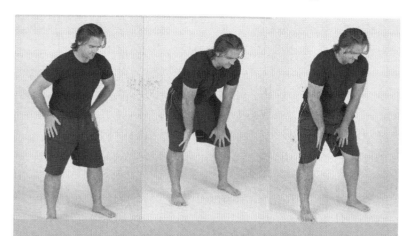

Glute and Hamstring Massage. With each hand, stroke from your buttocks downward across the back of your thighs and ending at the back of the inside of your knees, and then return with a stroke upward along your outer thigh ending at your buttock.

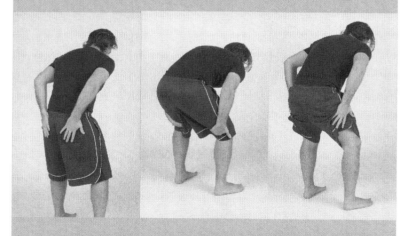

Lower Leg Massage. With each hand, stroke from the back of your knees downward across your calves to your ankles, and then return with a stroke upward along the front of your shin.

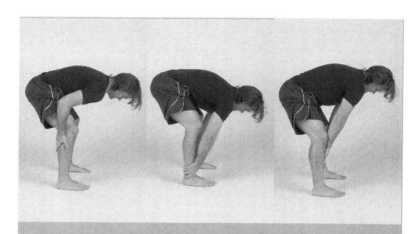

Foot Massage. With your right hand under the front of your right foot reaching from the outside and with your left hand under the back of your right foot reaching from the inside, stroke each hand out from under your right foot, your right hand moving to the right and your left hand moving to the left. With your hands reversed, repeat this for your left foot.

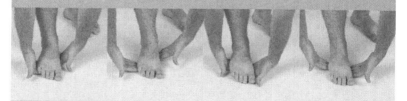

This simple self-massage routine will help to prepare your body for exercise.

The second component of a warm-up is the general warm-up, which smooths the major motions of the body, making the entire body swell and sweat, preparing it for the workout. One of the first things that needs to happen in a workout is a sweat that spreads over the whole body. Galen explains what a warm-up should be: "... preparatory exercise in quantity of movements is not more than moderate, and in quality more intense and quicker"[72] so it thereby warms, constricts, and contracts the body, removing relaxation and making the body strong and ready for action. The speed and strength of the movements prepare the body to work hard.

Preparatory Movements

There are many legitimate ways to warm-up. Walking and jogging both work very well. The following is a useful routine requiring no equipment which should work for almost everyone. With all of these preparatory exercises, start slowly and build the speed of the movement as it feels comfortable and smooth. The length of time this warm-up will take and the number of repetitions to do will vary by person and by the season. Some people have naturally warm legs but naturally cold arms, or vice versa, and during the cold times of the year it will take longer to warm the body compared to the hot times of the year.

Heel Raises. Raise yourself to your tiptoes and lower yourself back down. Start slowly and build to a quick movement once it is comfortable and smooth. Your ankles, heels, and calves should feel warm by the time you stop.

---

72 Hygiene, p133.

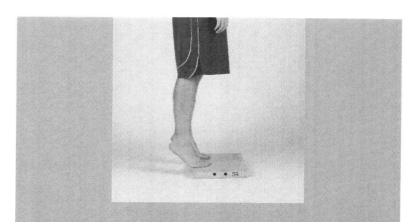

Deep Knee Bends. Bend your knees while raising up on your toes and then return to standing. Start slowly and build to a quick movement once it is comfortable and smooth. Your knees and thighs should feel warm by the time you stop.

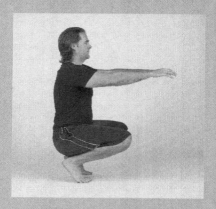

Reach and Bends. Reach up to the sky with your arms and look up with your head, and then bend forward, aiming to touch your toes. Repeat this movement many times. Start slowly and build to a quick movement once it is comfortable and smooth. Add range as you feel warm, leaning backward at the top and aiming to place your hands deeper toward the floor. Your hamstrings, spine, abdomen, shoulders, and neck should feel warm before you stop.

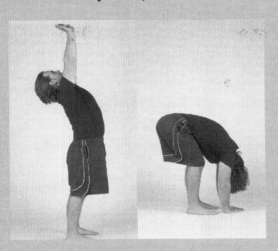

Standing Trunk Twist. With your arms straight out to your sides, twist your trunk so that your chest and arms turn to the left while your pelvis and head both stay facing forward, then reverse the movement to turn to the right. Repeat slowly and build to a quick movement once it is comfortable and smooth. Your spine, shoulders, and neck should feel warm by the time you stop.

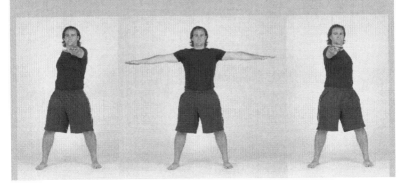

Shoulder Circles. With your arms straight out to your sides, make small circles forward and backward with your hands. When your shoulders feel warm, increase the size of these circles until you are making large circles with your shoulders. Start slowly and build to a quick movement once it is smooth and comfortable. Your shoulders and neck should feel warm before you stop.

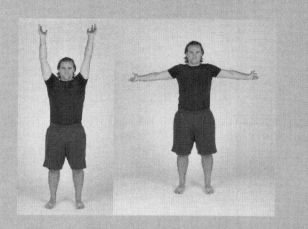

Easy Push-ups. With your hands elevated to such a height that you could perform at least 30 push-ups without grunting, perform push-ups. Start slowly and build to a quick movement once it is comfortable and smooth. Your shoulders, upper arms, elbows, forearms, and hands should feel warm before you stop.

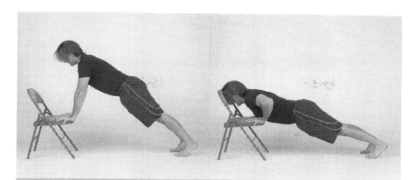

Burpees. From a push-up position, leap your feet forward so that you are in a squat position and then perform a jump. Upon landing from the jump, place your hands on the floor while returning to a squat position and leap your feet back to the push-up position. Repeat this movement many times, increasing the height of the jump, the length of the leap, and the speed of the entire movement as it feels comfortable and smooth. Take rest breaks as necessary to prevent yourself from overworking your muscles and from panting heavily, and stop once you've built up a sweat.

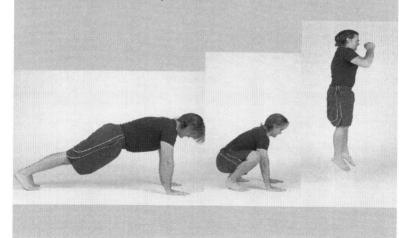

This sequence of gentle exercises will warm your entire body and get you sweating, preparing you effectively for a workout.

The third component of a warm-up is the specific warm-up, that is, preparing the body to perform the exercises that it will perform in the workout. If we are to run, then we start by gently running and build from there as the motion of running becomes smooth and fluid. If we are to do squats, then we start with light, easy squats, and add weight as the movement feels smooth and natural. The specific warm-up will be unique to the actual workout we will perform.

Each of these three components to a warm-up are vitally important to properly prepare the body for the workout proper.

The Workout Proper

The workout proper is the vigorous, swift, and violent exercises that we use to warm, dry, strengthen, and expel waste. We should be sweating by the time our preparatory movements are complete. This sweat should continue through the workout proper. The workout proper is essentially our way of ensuring that we expel our waste and keep our bodies strong by grunting and panting. Weightlifting gets us grunting, and running gets us panting. As long as we mildly challenge ourselves by grunting and panting, and as long as we sweat enough to expel our waste, the workout proper will be a success. We also need to ensure that we don't overdo it and cause injury or fatigue. The key is to work hard enough to grunt and pant, but gentle enough to not get hurt, and to work long enough to sweat a lot, but not so long as to get fatigued.

There is actually a large amount of wiggle-room for most people. Different exercises and ways of programming them affect our balance, so the workout proper must be properly done in order to balance the body.

We need to understand that all exercise is heating and drying; it's only a matter of how heating and drying a particular form of exercise is. So if we are in need of cooling or moistening, exercise is not our tool of choice. It can only be modified so as to be as minimally heating and drying as possible. The faster the exercise, the more heating it is.[73] Fast exercise, such as running, is very heating, while slow exercise, such as weightlifting, is less so.[74] The longer we exercise, the more drying it is.[75] The longer the workout, the longer the run, the more sets of an exercise we do, and the more repetitions we do per set, all make our exercise more drying. So if we are going to run, the longer we run, the more drying it is. Running 400m is more drying than running 200m.[76] Long distance running is much more drying than short distance running. The longer the total time of our workout, the more drying it will be. In addition, the rest breaks we take during our workout can make it more or less drying. The fewer and the shorter the rest breaks that we take between exercises, the more drying will be the workout.[77] Taking few or even no rest breaks between exercises encourages much sweating and is best for

---

73 Hippocrates 4, Regimen 1, Ch 35.
74 Hygiene, p195-6.
75 Hygiene, p195-6.
76 Hippocrates 4, Regimen 2, Ch 63.
77 Hygiene, p135.

those who are too moist. Taking frequent and long breaks between exercises helps to keep us from sweating much and is thus a good choice for those who are too dry. A person who is too dry and who is thus taking longer rest breaks should strive to get a sweat going, but then slow down in an attempt to keep the sweat from becoming profuse. Basically, the more we sweat, the more drying the workout is. To minimize the drying effects, we would want to do shorter workouts, shorter runs, less sets of exercises, less repetitions per set, and take longer rest breaks. The following chart helps to illustrate these effects.

	Slow Exercise	**Fast Exercise**
Large Amount	Mildly heating, very drying	Very heating, very drying
Moderate Amount	Mildly heating, moderately drying	Very heating, moderately drying
Small Amount	Mildly heating, mildly drying	Very heating, mildly drying

The chart helps us to control how our exercise affects our balance on the wobble board of health and helps to make our decisions about exercise fairly simple. If we're hot and moist, then a lot of slow exercise is best, drying us significantly but only mildly adding heat. If we're hot and dry, then a small amount of slow exercise is best, only mildly heating and drying us. If we're cold and dry, then a small amount of fast exercise is best, heating us a lot without drying us much. And if we are cold and moist, then a large amount of fast exercise is best, adding much heat and drying us significantly. But these are extreme examples. Galen says that "... the best condition of the body requires neither fast nor slow exercise, but intermediate and moderate; and in the same way neither vigorous and violent nor sluggish and weak, but again moderation is best."[78] This is very important. We should all default to a moderate amount of exercise. The length of our runs, the number of repetitions, and our rest breaks should all be moderate unless we have good reason to do otherwise.

If we are grunting by five repetitions, then we're using a large amount of resistance, and if we aren't grunting until about 15 repetitions, then we're using a small amount of resistance. A good moderate average between these two extremes is ten repetitions. So our default way to exercise should be to aim to be grunting by ten repetitions. Similarly, a moderate way to run would be somewhere between the fast speed of a sprint and the slow speed of a jog. To pant from running 100m requires one to run very fast, essentially to sprint, and in order to not be panting from a run that is longer than one mile (1600m), one would need to jog very slowly. Moderate distances for a run range from 200m to one mile, making us pant while running at a reasonable pace. The following chart illustrates these effects:

	Effect	Reps/Set	Run
Long	Very drying	15	>1600m
Moderate	Drying	10	200-1600m
Short	Mildly drying	5	<200m

78 Hygiene, p92.

The ancient Greeks elevated the 200m run (a half-lap around a modern track) to the highest level. It was the primary event at the Olympics, the winner of which was crowned victor of the Olympic games, with the next four years named after him. Hippocrates follows suit. He uses 200m and 400m as his primary examples of running distances, with 200m being considered the default, and 400m being considered a long run. This is a really important thing to consider. In the modern world, we think of long runs as marathons, while ancient people considered a long run to be one lap around a modern track. Short distance running is sprinting less than 200m, and long-distance running is running anything more than one mile. We should start considering running more than one mile to be a very long-distance run. Dr. Cooper's 1968 book entitled *Aerobics*, which in some ways started the aerobic fitness revolution, recommended running one sub-eight-minute mile per day for those who were already in shape to maintain their fitness.[79] Somehow we went from running one mile to running marathons, following the obviously fallacious concept that if *some* is good, then *more* must be better. Most people should stick to the middle range, running 200m if they are on the dry side, and 400m if they are on the moist side. For very moist people at very moist times, perhaps a mile run or even more is appropriate, but this is only for extreme situations.

We should also default to using rest breaks that are moderate, neither rushed nor so slow as to potentially lose our flush and sweat. The moderate rest break is to start the

---

79 Cooper. *Aerobics*. New York: Bantam Books, 1968. P20 of The Aerobics Point System insert.

next exercise as soon as one's breathing begins to return to the state it was before the previous exercise.

Rest Breaks	Amount of Sweat
Short or none - rushed	Lots - very drying
Moderate	Significant - drying
Long	Minimal - mild drying

There are other effects of exercise to take into consideration. Galen says, "... much exercise [thins] the body, and moderate exercise fattens it, or puts on flesh."[80] Doing a large amount of exercise melts our flesh and leaves us thinner, which is useful for those who are overfat. A moderate amount of exercise does the opposite, building our flesh, which is useful for those who are too thin. And a small amount of exercise does nothing to either add or subtract flesh from our bodies, which makes it an appropriate amount of exercise for those who are neither too lean nor too fat.

We define a little amount of exercise as one set taken to the point when the body is flushed and challenged, when the performance of the exercise would be less smooth if continued. A moderate amount of exercise is three sets taken to the point of being challenged, and a lot of exercise is five sets taken to the beginning of deviating from smooth motion. We should never push ourselves beyond the point at which our movement is smooth and controlled. This is true for both

---

80 Hygiene, p196.

resistance exercises and for running. The following chart summarizes:

Amount of Exercise	Sets	Effect on Flesh
Much	Five runs or sets	Melts flesh
Moderate	Three runs or sets	Builds flesh
Little	One run or set	No effect

So if we do lots of walking, running, or weightlifting, then we will end up with less flesh. If we do a moderate amount of these, then we will build some flesh. And if we do a little, we will not add or subtract flesh.

We discussed earlier how vigorous exercise, the kind that makes us grunt, strengthens the body. It also hardens the body. The more vigorous our exercise, the more hardening is the effect. So a body that is too soft benefits from vigorous exercise, while a body that is too hard will become even more imbalanced by such exercise. We can harden the body by using less repetitions when doing vigorous exercise, closer to five repetitions per set, and we can prevent further hardening by using higher repetitions, closer to fifteen repetitions. The following chart summarizes:

Repetitions per Set	Effect
15 repetitions per set	Not hardening
10 repetitions per set	Slightly hardening
5 repetitions per set	Very hardening

The major way that Galen classifies exercises is based on swift versus slow, and vigorous versus non-vigorous. He says, "... some [exercises] produce slow movements, and some swift movements, and some vigorously, and some atonically...."[81] This gives us the following four categories of exercises:

- Gentle Exercises: are exercises that are neither swift nor vigorous and include such things as walking, stretching, and light calisthenics;
- Swift Exercises: are not vigorous enough to make us grunt, but fast enough to make us pant, the primary example being running;
- Vigorous Exercises: are vigorous in that they require us to work hard enough to grunt while we do them, the primary example being weightlifting and other resistance exercises; and
- Violent Exercises: are both swift and vigorous, including such exercises as explosive weightlifting, throwing the discus, and running while pushing a heavy sled.

This gives us the following chart:

81 Hygiene, p82.

	Vigorous	**Non-Vigorous**
Swift	Violent Exercise such as explosive lifting	Swift Exercise such as running
Slow	Vigorous Exercise such as weight-lifting	Gentle Exercise such as walking

Each type of exercise is appropriate for different needs. Gentle forms of exercise are those exercises that barely make us breathe harder or faster. The most obvious example is walking, but both our preparatory exercises and our apotherapeutic exercises (which we'll discuss soon) are also forms of gentle exercise. Gentle exercises are slow, so they do not generate much heat, and because they don't require much force, they can be done for prolonged periods of time. This makes gentle exercises useful for those who are too moist because they can be done for a long time in order to help to dry the body. Gentle exercises lend themselves to those who are hot and moist by allowing these people to exercise for a long period of time in order to dry the body without adding significant amounts of heat.

Gentle exercises are the most versatile of exercises. They warm without excessively heating. They can safely be used for long or short periods of time. They carry little risk of injury or fatigue because they require little force and little speed.

Walking is Hippocrates' favorite form of exercise, and deserves a special discussion because of its importance.

Walking is different from other forms of exercise because it is considered a Natural Exercise, that is, it is something the body does naturally such as seeing, hearing, thinking, and feeling. For this reason, walking is not considered a workout and doesn't require a warm-up or a cool-down. Along with apotherapy, it is unique in this way. All the other forms of exercise that we'll discuss require a warm-up and a cool-down, and walking can be a form of both warm-up and cool-down for other exercises.

Hippocrates says that there are three good times to walk:[82]

1. In the early morning,
2. After a workout, and
3. After a meal.

In the early morning, walking helps to gently warm the body for the day's activities and gets the bowels to function smoothly. After a workout, walking, like apotherapy, helps to purge waste material from the body and thus prevents fatigue and injuries. After a meal, walking dries the belly, preventing the gaining of belly fat and aiding digestion. One of the major uses of walking is to gently warm and dry the body, and expel waste, while risking very little in the way of injury.

Swift exercises are those that require us to move fast enough that our rate of breathing significantly increases. The most obvious examples are running, swimming, hiking, jumping rope, and biking. Swift exercises are fast, so they generate a lot of heat, and because they don't require much force, they

---

82 Hippocrates 4, Regimen 2, Ch 62.

can be done for prolonged periods of time, so they can be used to dry us significantly. Swift exercise is the most heating and drying form of exercise. It is best for those who are cold and moist, and it can be imbalancing for those who are hot and/or dry.

Swift Exercise, such as running, can be performed at such a fast rate that they actually become Violent Exercise because of the force required to perform them, and they can be performed at such a slow rate that they become Gentle Exercise because they are no longer swift enough to be considered Swift Exercise. For example, a 40-yard dash is so fast and requires such vigorous force that it should be considered Violent Exercise. Similarly, running so slowly that it should properly be called a jog is not really swift enough to be considered Swift Exercise. Jogging is best considered a slow Swift Exercise, or a swift Gentle Exercise, more on the cusp between Gentle Exercise and Swift Exercise than belonging to either category. Any run beyond one mile is closer to a jog than a run, and certainly anything more than three miles cannot be considered swift exercise.

Vigorous exercises are slow exercises that require enough force to perform that they make us grunt or hold our breath, but they don't require speed to perform. Galen defines them: "... I call a vigorous exercise one which exercises forcibly without speed...."[83] The most obvious examples are the basic barbell lifts: the deadlift, squat, overhead press, and row. Calisthenics can also be a vigorous form of exercise if done in

---

83 Hygiene, p82.

a way that requires one to grunt. Examples include push-ups, bar dips, chin-ups, and leaping.

Vigorous exercises have a very equivalent effect on our balance as do gentle exercises in that they are slow and so do not generate a lot of heat. The main difference between gentle exercise and vigorous exercise is the use of force. This use of force makes vigorous exercises more likely to cause us injury, specifically Tension Fatigue, and it also makes vigorous exercises much less versatile than gentle exercises because although one can easily walk for a long period of time, it would be almost impossible and certainly injurious to lift weights for a prolonged period of time. The main reason to use vigorous exercise is to strengthen the body.

Violent exercises are those exercises that are both swift and vigorous. Galen defines them: "... I call ... a violent exercise one which exercises forcibly with speed...."[84] These are exercises that are done with speed against a significant resistance. The most obvious examples are the explosive lifts: the clean, the jerk, and the snatch. Throwing the discus, running with a weight vest or while pushing a heavy object, and repeated jumping are ancient examples of violent exercises.[85]

The speed of violent exercises makes them significantly heating to the body, but because they require a great deal of force, making them difficult to perform for prolonged periods of time, they are not the most drying of exercises. Therefore,

---

84 Hygiene, p82.
85 Hygiene, p86.

violent forms of exercise are best for those who are cold and dry.

It's important to note that although the elderly are those most in need of heat and moisture, and therefore violent exercises may seem like a good choice for the elderly because they heat without drying much, violent exercise is not a good choice for the elderly. Galen and Hippocrates both make clear that violent exercises, because they are the most dangerous of all exercises, are not a good choice for the elderly. So violent exercise is best for those young people who are too cold and too dry.

Violent exercises are the most dangerous and the least versatile of exercises. One can only throw a discus quickly. There is no slow way to throw it. The lack of versatility of these exercises is a major drawback. Squats can be done both quickly or slowly. One can power walk or meander. One can run quickly or slowly. All the other types of exercise give us options. The violent ones do not.

Violent exercises are the most likely to cause injury and Tension Fatigue because of the force and speed required to perform them. The benefit of violent exercises is that, if performed wisely, they make us strong and powerful and less likely to be injured by daily life. Violent exercises are the most effective and efficient forms of exercise. They make us faster and stronger at the same time. So violent exercise is both the most useful form of exercise for preventing injury and the most likely form of exercise to cause injury. They're dangerous but useful.

Obviously, different exercises work different parts of the body. Galen says that running and walking work the legs, shadow-boxing works the arms, bending forward and backward, deadlifting, and supporting something continuously with the arms works the loins, and deep breathing and phonation works the lungs and thorax.[86] We want to ensure that we exercise our entire body in a balancing way, so we need at least a few exercises in our workout, at least one for each part of the body.

The following comment from Galen must be taken into consideration: "Rowing, digging, reaping, spear-throwing, running, jumping, riding, hunting, and armed combat - the natural performance of all these activities is preferable to exercise in the gymnasium."[87] Basically, whenever possible, we should attempt to find ways to get our exercise from our daily lives. If we spend 45 minutes digging up a tree stump, then there's no reason to do any other workout for the day. Whenever possible such activities should replace our workouts. The workout proper is not the ideal, it's just a necessity in the lives of those who are not very active in their daily lives. We only need to do the major movements, and then we should call it a day. And ideally we live our lives so that there is rarely a need to do a workout because we do enough vigorous and strenuous things to grunt, pant, and sweat in our daily lives. But the reality of most of our lives is that we simply aren't physically active enough and so need a workout to help us to stay balanced.

---

86 Hygiene. P87.
87 Selected. P92.

There are an infinite number of ways to put together a reasonable workout regimen that effectively and safely makes us grunt, pant, and sweat. The following regimen keeps the workout proper very simple. It will prove effective for most people.

The Workout Proper

Run. Run a balancing distance at a pace that makes you pant, and repeat this a balancing number of times with a balancing rest break between each run. An alternative is to use burpees, jumping rope, swimming, biking, hill hiking, or stair climbing. It takes about 30 seconds to 2 minutes to run 400m, which is the basic moderate distance for most people to run. So each set of these other exercises should take approximately that length of time at a pace that makes you pant. Walking up a hill is perhaps the gentlest way to pant and sweat, risking very little in the way of injuries and maximizing the effect. Hiking hills and stairs are both very useful and safe swift exercises that include panting and sweating without a large risk of injury. It is the downhill part of hiking and it is the downward motion on the stairs that is most likely to cause injury, so the best way is to hike up a steep hill and then down a gentle grade, and to go up steps and then find another way to come down. At the very least, one can just go slowly down the hill or stairs, using the upward part of the climb as the exercise and the downward part as the rest.

Push-ups. Do push-ups with your hands or feet elevated so that a set of a balancing number of repetitions makes you grunt. Push-ups are an excellent exercise for almost everyone. There are few people who can't safely and effectively use push-ups. You can elevate your hands as high as necessary in order to make the push-ups easy enough to perform. If you are very strong, you can elevate your feet as high as necessary to make them challenging, even to the point of doing handstand push-ups. An excellent alternative is to perform overhead presses with a barbell or to do bar dips. Pull-ups and rows are also excellent upper body exercises that involve a pulling motion of the upper body instead of the pushing motion of push-ups. It is ideal to divide your upper body sets among a pushing exercise and a pulling exercise. If you are going to do three sets of upper body exercises, then you could do two sets of push-ups and one set of pull-ups, for example.

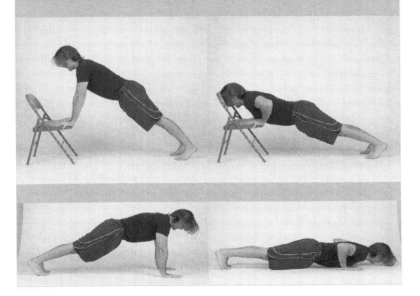

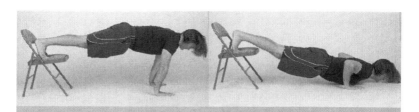

Deadlifts. Stand over a weight, bend down at the hips keeping your back straight, grab the weight, and stand back up. This is a deadlift. It is one of the most ancient of all exercises and works just about the entire body. Alternatives include squats, single leg squats, and long jumping. To do a set of long jumps, simply jump forward for a balancing number of repetitions far enough that you must grunt by the end of the set. The long jump is recommended instead of the vertical jump because the force of landing from a vertical jump, which can easily be more than ten times the force of landing from a long jump, dramatically increases the risk of injury. Nevertheless, vertical jumps are also a reasonable alternative exercise. It is totally acceptable to split the sets of lower body exercises amongst a couple of exercises, doing perhaps two sets of deadlifts and one set of long jumps.

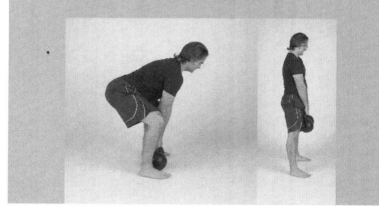

It is highly recommended (perhaps 'required' is a better word choice) to run and jump on a soft surface such as grass. Running or jumping on concrete or asphalt is asking for (or demanding) an injury.

These three simple exercises, running, push-ups, and deadlifts, and their alternatives, make an excellent workout routine for almost everyone.

Apotherapy

"Apotherapy is called the final part of all well-completed exercise."[88] - Galen

Apotherapy is how we end our workouts. It consists of alternating between massage and stretches performed slowly and gently to cool and calm the body after the hard work of the workout.[89] Apotherapeutic exercises are relaxing, reducing the tension of the workout proper. Galen explains them: "... the so-called apotherapeutic exercises, in which it is possible also to make movements, moderate in quantity and slow in quality, with many pauses between them, in which the man must be massaged... in order that the excrements might be eliminated as quickly as possible."[90]

Apotherapy helps to prevent fatigue. Basically, the massage and stretching of apotherapy help to expel waste materials that were created by the workout. Apotherapy helps to ensure

---

88 Hygiene, p101.
89 Hygiene, p103, p105.
90 Hygiene, p118.

that we don't get Ulcerous Fatigue. And the massage helps to soften any muscles that have hardened from excessive force during exercise, making it less likely that we will develop Tension Fatigue. Apotherapy is insurance against fatigue.

Exercise warms and thins the waste material in the body, and sweating and breathing during the workout helps to get some of them out, but much of the excrement still remains in the body after exercise. Massage, stretching, and compression of the breath all work to squeeze out the waste. Stretching helps expel waste by forcing them out as an internal massage against the skin. It's important to keep the intent in mind: we aren't stretching to gain range of motion, but to squeeze waste out of the tissues. So very gentle is the name of the game for apotherapeutic stretches.

Health abhors sudden change, so it is important that the body does not cool too rapidly after exercise. It is often a good idea to wrap oneself in a blanket during apotherapy to help to slow the cooling of the body, making it a gradual cooling. Shivering is a sign of a sudden change from hot to cold. When we exercise, we warm the body, and the body flushes and sweats in order to cool itself. If we exercise too hard, too long, or in too cool of a place, then the body can easily cool itself too much, causing us to shiver. And when we stop exercising, the sweat can quickly cause us to shiver. We must always remember that sudden changes are what can easily throw us off balance into disease. Shivering is a dangerous sign that we did not maintain our balance. There are four things we must do in order to prevent shivering when we exercise. First, we must make sure that we exercise in a comfortable place that won't cool us too quickly. Second, we must watch ourselves to ensure that we stop exercising whenever our bodies begin to lose the flush and sweat that are natural parts of exercise. The loss of the flush and the sweat is a sign that we have pushed ourselves too hard or too long. Third, we need to take the time to cool down gradually after exercising. That is, we must not stop suddenly, but do gentle movements and exercises to end our workout, such as apotherapy. Fourth, we should often wrap ourselves in extra clothing at the end of a workout in order to slow the heat loss due to sweating. It's best to exercise as close to nude as possible (the ancient Greeks exercised naked) in order to allow the body to cool itself efficiently when exercising, and then to wrap up in some clothing immediately upon stopping exercise in order to prevent too rapid of cooling.

The following is a simple apotherapeutic routine that is appropriate for almost everyone.

Apotherapy

Deep Squats. Keeping your feet flat on the floor, squat down as deeply as you comfortably can. If you must, hang onto a sturdy object as you do this. Repeat about ten times to pump fluid through your legs and trunk.

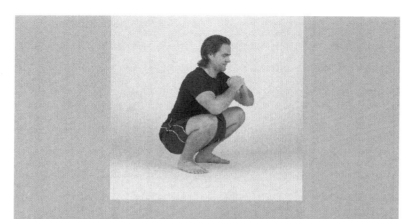

Shoulder Rolls. Roll your shoulder blades forward and backward in a smooth and relaxed manner. Repeat about ten times in each direction. The idea is to reduce tension in the shoulder and neck muscles.

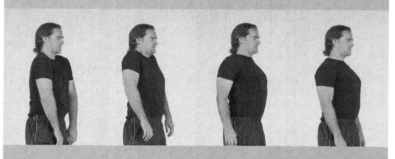

Massage Neck and Arms. Perform the neck, shoulder, lat and pec, arms, and hand massage techniques from the preparatory massage routine. By default, use a moderate amount of pressure and a short duration (perhaps five strokes of the hand) for apotherapeutic massage.

Neck Stretches. With your right hand behind your back, stretch your neck by dropping your nose to your left armpit and using your left hand to add some gentle pressure to this stretch. Repeat this to the other side. Then, with your left hand behind your back, stretch your neck by lifting your nose away from your left armpit. Repeat this to the other side also. Hold each stretch for about ten seconds.

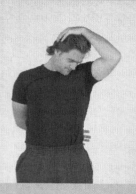
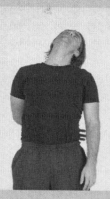

Tricep and Lat Stretch. Reach your right hand behind your upper back and use your left hand to gently pull your right elbow backward and to the left. This will stretch your right lat and tricep. Hold it for about ten seconds, and then repeat on the other side.

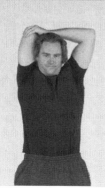

Upper Back Stretch. Reach your right arm across your body and use your left arm to gently pull your right upper arm across your body to stretch your right upper back and shoulder muscles. Hold this stretch for about ten seconds, and then repeat on the other side.

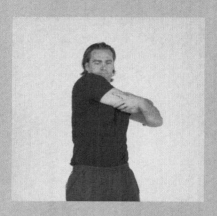

Bicep and Pec Stretch. Interlace the fingers of your hands behind your back and, with your elbows straight, lift your hands as high as you can to gently stretch your chest and biceps. Hold this stretch for about ten seconds.

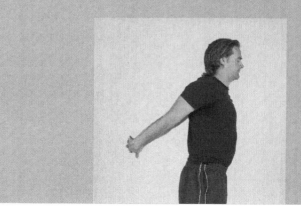

Forearm Stretches. With the point of your right elbow pointing straight down to the ground, with the elbow kept straight, and with the palm of your right hand turned down toward the ground, use your left hand to bend your wrist toward the ground to stretch the back of your forearm. Hold this for about ten seconds. Then, with your elbow still straight and pointing to the ground, turn your palm upward and then use your left hand to bend your right wrist downward to stretch the inside of your forearm muscles. Hold this for ten seconds, and then switch to stretch the inside and outside of your left forearm muscles.

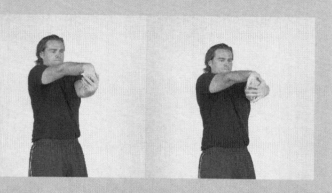

Finger Stretches. With your elbows straight, interlace your fingers and spread them to stretch the palms and fingers of your hands.

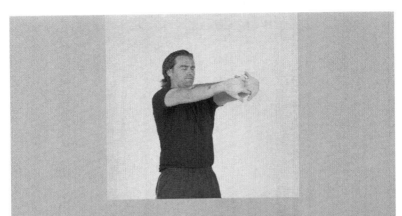

Breath Compressions. Stand with your hands behind your neck, take a deep breath and hold it, then use your hands to gently pull your chin to your chest and round your mid-back, keeping your abdomen relaxed. It will feel as if your upper abdomen is expanding and stretching. Hold your breath and the position for as long as you comfortably can, and then exhale and return to the starting position. Repeat three times. These Breath Compression help to expel waste from your lungs, helping to fully complete the cleansing effects of exercise, and helping to prevent the coughing and lung irritation that can often result from exercise.[91]

---

91 Hygiene, p104.

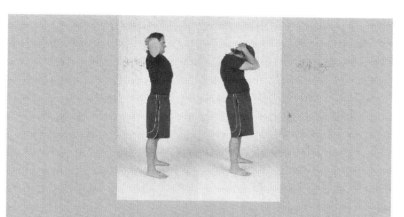

Standing Thigh Stretch. Use both hands to pull your right ankle to your buttock to stretch the front of your right thigh. Hold the stretch for ten seconds and then repeat on the other side.

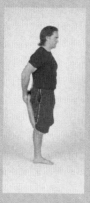

Hip Flexor Stretch. Stand in a lunge position with your right leg behind you and with your right arm reached up in the air, and then lunge forward into your left leg to gently stretch the front of your right hip. Hold this stretch for ten seconds and then repeat on the other side.

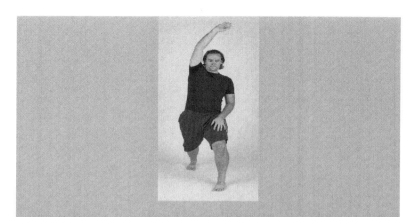

Shin Stretch. Place the top of your right toes against the ground to stretch the front of your right shin muscles. Hold for ten seconds and then repeat on the other side.

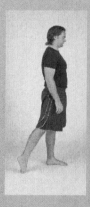

Calf Stretch. Place the bottom of your right toes against a wall to stretch your right calf muscle. Hold for ten seconds and then repeat on the other side. The Downward Dog pose from yoga is a good alternative.

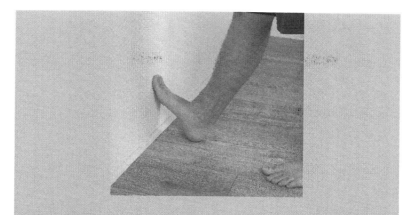

Cobra Stretch. Assume a quadruped position and then drop your pelvis forward to arch your back. Hold this stretch for ten seconds.

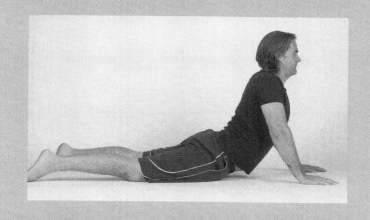

Child's Stretch. From a quadruped position, bend your knees to bring your buttocks toward your heels. This will mildly stretch your low back. Hold this stretch for ten seconds.

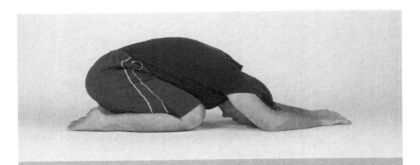

Foot Stretch. Sit on your ankles with your toes extended on the ground to stretch the bottom of your feet. Hold this stretch for ten seconds.

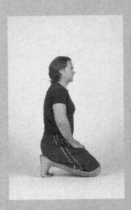

Side-Lying Trunk, Low Back, and Glute Massage and Trunk Twist Stretch. Lie on your left side with your knees bent comfortably, using a pillow to ensure that your neck is comfortable. Use your right hand to massage the inner part of your right thigh, the front part of your right thigh, the back and outside of your right thigh, the front of your right hip, your right buttock, and the right side of your lower back and pelvis. Use your left hand to massage the right side of your ribs and armpit. When you've finished massaging, rotate your trunk to the right to stretch your trunk, keeping your knees on the ground by anchoring them with your left hand. Hold this stretch for ten seconds. Repeat all of this on the opposite side.

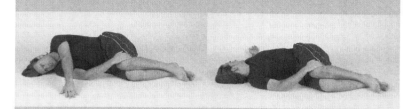

Adductor Stretch. Lie face up and bring your knees up toward your chest and outward to the sides, stretching your inner thighs. Hold this stretch for ten seconds.

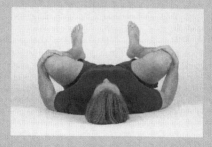

Hip Stretches. Pull your right knee to your chest and hold for ten seconds. Rest the outside of your right ankle on your left lower thigh and gently pull your right knee toward your left chest to stretch the back of your right hip. Hold this for ten seconds. Hold your right thigh vertical and straighten your right knee to stretch your hamstrings. Hold this stretch for ten seconds.

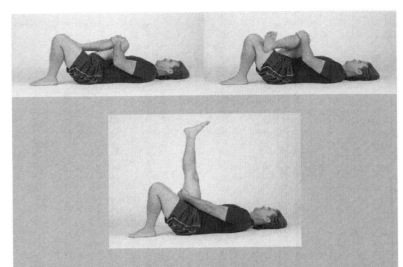

Calf, Shin, and Foot Massage. From the above position, use both hands to massage your right calf and shin, and the bottom of your right foot.

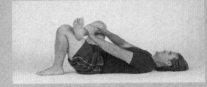

Repeat the hip stretches and lower body massage on the left side.

Apotherapy is a form of gentle exercise and it may sometimes be the only form of exercise worth doing. On days in which one is fatigued and needs a rest from exercise, apotherapy may be all that one does. The daily massaging and stretching of apotherapy can be wonderfully balancing for the body. These things alone heat the body, soften it, and help to expel waste, which are the primary reasons that we exercise.

A complete workout is three phases: preparing the body adequately, the workout proper, and apotherapy. We've discussed the details of each and how to make it balancing for each individual's need.

Constitutional and Seasonal Exercise

In order for exercise to be balancing for one's health, it must balance the effects of one's constitution and the season. Those who are hot by nature should make slow exercises their default selection. Resistance exercises and walking should be the staple of their exercise routine. Swift exercises, such as running and explosive lifting, are not totally out of the question, but they should only be done if living in a cool place or during the cooler months of the year. In contrast, those who are cold by nature can choose from all types of exercise, because all exercise is warming, but should emphasize swift exercises, such as running, for most of the year. If living in a hot place or during the hottest months of the year, these people can probably run less or even not at all, but the rest of the year should be devoted to swifter exercise.

Those who are dry by nature should do only small amounts of exercise, especially during the dry times of the year and especially if living in a dry place. During the moist time of year or if living in a moist place, these people can tolerate a bit more exercise, but they should always error toward less. Those who are moist by nature can tolerate and benefit from much exercise, especially during the moist months of the year. During the dry time of year or if living in a dry place, these people can get away with a little less exercise, but most of the year they need to be doing longer amounts of exercise. Any type of exercise will do, but since it should be done for a longer duration, the best choice is the less vigorous forms of exercise that allow them to continue to exercise for long periods of time, such as walking and running.

Those who are hot and moist should do longer amounts of slow exercise in order to dry while avoiding excessive heating. This can be done with lots of walking, or with longer sessions of higher repetition resistance exercise. During the cold and dry months, these people can get away with a bit of swift, heating exercise and with a bit shorter bouts of exercise, but in general they need lots of slow exercise. These people have a major challenge: they must exercise to help them to not be too moist, but they must avoid getting too hot. This is a difficult challenge, for it is all too easy to end up with excessive heat from exercising, and yet without exercising the moisture can easily get out of hand. Walking is a wonderful form of exercise for these people. It allows them to get lots of exercise without risking much heat. Walking done in the cool of the morning or in the cover of the evening is their best bet, especially during the hot times of the year.

Those who are hot and dry need to be careful not to overdo exercise. These people need exercise the least of all people. A small amount of slow, vigorous exercise, such as resistance exercise, can be taken, especially during the cooler months or if they live in a cold place, but these people should always error on the side of less. These people can often get away with almost no exercise, especially if they live in a hot and dry place and especially during the hot and dry months of the year. A short, gentle walk may be all that they need, and maybe all that they can tolerate in order to stay healthy.

Those who are cold and dry should do short bouts of swift, warming exercises, such as running or explosive lifting to warm without getting too dry. These people will benefit from a few short runs and from short weightlifting sessions. These people have a major challenge: they must exercise to warm themselves, but they must avoid getting too dry. Fortunately, all they must do is keep their exercise sessions short in order to avoid trouble.

Those who are cold and moist have the easiest time selecting an exercise plan. They simply need exercise, and lots of it. They will benefit most from longer sessions of swift, heating exercises. The most obvious form of exercise for these people is long distance running. These people simply need lots of exercise in any form, since all exercise is heating and drying. This is especially true during the cold and moist months and even more true if these people live in a cold place. If these people live in hot places, and during the hot months of the year, they may be able to tolerate less exercise, but they'd be wise to at least consistently take swift, long walks to maintain their heat and to keep from getting too moist.

We also need to adjust our workouts with the changing weather patterns through the year. As we adjust through the year, we need to adjust slowly. In the hot and dry months we take less exercise, and in the cold and moist months we take more. We therefore should be slowly ramping up our exercise during the cold and dry months, and slowly decreasing our exercise during the hot and moist months. Everyone's year should go something like the following. In the cold and moist months we are doing the most exercise that we will do all year. We are doing relatively long workouts of the swiftest exercises that we'll do all year. A cold and moist person living in a cold and moist place may be running very long distances during the cold and moist months. A hot and dry person living in a hot and dry place may only be walking long distances in the cool of the early morning or late afternoon and doing a short weightlifting session at this time.

In the hot and moist months, we should all be decreasing our exercise, preparing for the hot and dry months to come. We will still be doing relatively long workouts to help us to stay dry, but with the increasing heat we will want to start doing slower exercises. Runs will start to become jogs, and jogs will become walks.

In the hot and dry months, we should all be doing the least exercise that we will do all year. Our workouts should be relatively short sessions of relatively slow exercises. A cold and moist person living in a cold and moist place may still be running during this time, but should be running shorter distances and going at a slower pace. A hot and dry person living in a hot and dry place should probably be almost not exercising at all, perhaps just doing a short walk in the cool of the morning and evening.

In the cold and dry months, we should all be increasing our exercise, preparing for the cold and moist months to come. Our workouts should still be short in order to avoid excessive drying, but we can begin to increase the swiftness. A cold and moist person would begin to run faster again, slowly increasing the distance over the season. A hot and dry person would be able to start exercising a bit more, doing short walks and short weightlifting sessions to prepare for the cold and moist months.

Planning Your Exercise Regimen

Putting this all together so that you can choose a workout plan for any given day can seem overwhelming. We need a strategy from which to plan your regimen. The best place to start is with your constitution.[92] That will help you plan the foundation for all of your workouts. From there, you can adjust for the basic weather pattern of the place in which you live, and then adjust for the current needs of any given day.

Get out your Constitutional and Seasonal Maps and refer to them as you read this section.

The best way to plan your personal workout program is to start by planning the workouts for the cold and moist months. The cold and moist months are when you can do the most exercise and the most extreme forms of it that your constitution will allow. Then you can plan the workouts for the hot and dry months, which will be the workouts with the least amount of exercise in its most gentle form. Then it becomes

92 Hygiene, p263.

easy to plan the rest of the year, which is just a gradual transition between these two extremes. In the hot and moist months you gradually decrease both the amount and the swiftness of your exercise, and in the cold and dry months you gradually increase both the amount and swiftness of your exercise.

We'll start with a well-balanced exercise routine appropriate for the cold and moist time of the year for a person with a well-balanced constitution: warm-up (as discussed earlier); workout proper (taking moderate rest breaks between each exercise and between each set): 1) Run 3x400m (three 400m runs), 2) Push-ups 3x10 (three sets of ten repetitions), and 3) Deadlifts 3x10; and then apotherapy (as discussed earlier).

The 400m run is heating and drying to balance the cold and moist weather of the season, and the push-ups and deadlifts are vigorous exercises that strengthen the entire body at a moderate range of repetitions, performed for three sets which helps to moderately dry the body during the moist season. This basic plan must be modified to meet one's constitutional needs. The following chart is helpful for this purpose:

	Cold	Moderate	Hot
Dry	Run 4x800m Lift 4x10	Run 4x400m Lift 4x10	Run 4x200m Lift 4x10
Moderate	Run 3x800m Lift 3x10	Run 3x400m Lift 3x10	Run 3x200m Lift 3x10
Moist (less drying)	Run 2x800m Lift 2x10	Run 2x400m Lift 2x10	Run 2x200m Lift 2x10

From this chart, start in the middle, which is a well-balanced, moderate regimen, and then adjust according to your constitutional needs. For example, a person with a cold and moist constitution would shift one square toward the hot and one square toward the dry, choosing to run 200m four times, and performing 4 sets of ten repetitions of the resistance exercises.

The chart above is also useful for adjusting the workout to meet the needs of your location. For example, if the cold and moist time of the year is not all that cold, perhaps because you don't live where it snows in the winter, then your regimen should be adjusted one square toward the cold side of the chart to balance the lack of cold in the weather.

Write your exercise program for the cold and moist time of the year near the cold and moist section of your Seasonal Map.

Next, you should select your workout for the hot and dry time of the year. The table below shows the moderate regimen which should be your default selection, and then adjust as you did above.

	Cold	Moderate	Hot
Dry	Run 2x400m Lift 2x10	Run 2x200m Lift 2x10	Run 2x100m Lift 2x10
Moderate	Run 1x400m Lift 1x10	Run 1x200m Lift 1x10	Run 1x100m Lift 1x10
Moist (less drying)	Walk Lift 1x10	Walk Lift 1x10	Run 1x100m Lift 1x10

The default, moderate program of running 200m once and doing one set of ten repetitions of push-ups and deadlifts, should be modified to meet your constitutional needs. Our cold and moist example person would start from the moderate middle square and then adjust one square toward the hot and one square toward the dry side, selecting to run 100m twice and 2 sets of ten repetitions of the resistance exercises.

Write your exercise program for the hot and dry time of the year near the hot and dry section of your Seasonal Map.

All that is left is to plan a smooth transition between these extremes. The following table is for the hot and moist time of the year:

	Cold	Moderate	Hot
Dry	Run 3x800m Lift 3x10	Run 3x400m Lift 3x10	Run 3x200m Lift 3x10
Moderate	Run 2x800m Lift 2x10	Run 2x400m Lift 2x10	Run 2x200m Lift 2x10
Moist (less drying)	Run 1x800m Lift 1x10	Run 1x400m Lift 1x10	Run 1x200m Lift 1x10

Our example person with a cold and moist constitution would choose to run 200m four times and do 3x10 for his resistance exercises.

Write your exercise program for the hot and moist time of the year near the hot and moist section of your Seasonal Map.

Finally, the following table can be used for the cold and dry time of the year:

	Cold	Moderate	Hot
Dry	Run 3x400m	Run 3x200m	Run 3x100m
	Lift 3x10	Lift 3x10	Lift 3x10
Moderate	Run 2x400m	Run 2x200m	Run 2x100m
	Lift 2x10	Lift 2x10	Lift 2x10
Moist (less	Run 1x400m	Run 1x200m	Run 1x100m
drying)	Lift 1x10	Lift 1x10	Lift 1x10

Our example person with a cold and moist constitution would choose to run 100m three times and do 3x10 for his resistance exercises.

Write your exercise program for the cold and dry time of the year near the cold and dry section of your Seasonal Map.

It's important to note how flexible this programming can be. There are many alternatives. Any endurance exercise can replace running. You can jump rope, swim, hike, or bike. You can do sets of burpees done to a pant. And many things can replace the push-ups and deadlifts. Overhead presses, chin-ups, bar dips, squats, and long jumps are all great alternative options. Also, many activities can be divided into the various categories. For example, hitting a tennis serve at maximal power is a vigorous exercise, sprinting from place to place on the tennis court to hit the ball is a swift exercise, and practicing your strokes in a controlled manner is a gentle exercise. Anyone involved in any sport or recreational activity can often use it to meet various exercise needs simply by emphasizing various components of the activity at certain times of the year. Of course, this also means that these activities can be imbalancing if performed without giving thought to your balancing needs.

Your Seasonal Map should now be complete with an exercise regimen appropriate to your needs.

The two keys to using workouts in a healthy way is take the time to assess the needs of the day, and to know how to modify the workout in order to meet those needs. The way to do this is to always ask, "What would Hippocrates say?" during the warm-up for a workout. While warming-up for a workout, we assess our balance. We ask ourselves how we are doing, how balanced we are. We note whether we are too hot, too cold, too dry, or too moist. We should have a planned workout ready to go, but we should always be ready to modify it for the needs of the day. As examples, if we've had a busy day, then we need to know how to reduce the workout, and if it's unseasonably cold, then we need to know how to make the workout more heating. If we're cold and stiff, then we need to make sure that the workout warms us, and if we're hot and limber, then we need to make certain that the workout doesn't overheat us. Our daily exercise regimen must address the needs of our balance.

If one is exhausted or has already been very active during the day, then less exercise should be taken that day. If one is feeling hot, then slower exercises should be substituted for swifter ones. For example, if one would normally run 200m but is feeling excessively hot, then one could take a walk instead. If one is feeling cold, then one should substitute swifter exercises for slower ones, running instead of walking.

If one is feeling dry, then one should do less exercise than normal, such as a 200m run instead of a 400m run, or two sets of the resistance exercises instead of three. If one is feeling moist, then one should do more exercise than normal, such as taking a longer walk than usual, running 400m instead of 200m, or doing four sets instead of three sets for the resistance exercises.

In all these modifications it is important to make small changes. If we need to shift to a more drying workout, then we shouldn't switch from running 200m to running a mile. That's way too large of a change. Instead, we shift from running 200m to 400m. Likewise, we don't shift from deadlifting 250# for five repetitions to deadlifting 150# for fifteen repetitions. Instead, we make smaller changes. A small adjustment goes a long way toward adjusting our balance on the wobble board. We must remember that we are balancing. A large push in any direction can cause significant loss of balance. This is even true of resting and of taking a day off from exercise. In most situations, it'd be better to do an easy, gentle workout than to stop 'cold turkey.' And the reverse is obviously true. We don't want to go from no exercise to lots of exercise in one large leap.

It's important to note that the regimen we've been constructing is only a rough plan. As we exercise through the year, we will need to modify this plan to meet our needs. Perhaps the cold and moist time of year is much colder than we thought and so we'll need to make our workout plan more heating, or perhaps we aren't as moist as we thought and fifteen repetitions per set is just too drying for us, so we'll have to switch to ten repetitions per set. The point is that this basic plan is almost certainly in at least some way inaccurate for our needs. We should not follow it blindly. Each year we should grow more and more wise about how to balance to the needs of our constitutions and the seasons.

It's extremely helpful to think of the workout proper as a time to get ourselves sweating, grunting, and panting enough to balance the body, whatever that may require. Sometimes this means lots of sweating or grunting or panting, and sometimes a little, depending on one's constitution, the season, and the needs of the day. We can grunt with low repetitions or with high repetitions, depending on our needs. We can pant from a long run, from a short run, or from a walk. Sweating is both cleansing by way of expelling waste through sweat, and drying by the moisture lost through sweat. We know that by expelling waste, sweat is very helpful for our health, but the drying effect of sweat can be either balancing or imbalancing, so we need to take care with this effect of exercise. Those who are too moist by nature and especially during the moist times of the year, can be greatly benefited by emphasizing exercises that cause lots of sweat. On the contrary, those who are dry by nature and especially during the dry times of the year, must take care to sweat for the cleansing effect without excessively sweating.

Since exercise should be done to balance the needs of the day, the best time to do a workout is at the end of the day, long after we've digested our food and before we eat our final meal for the day, and after we've finished our activity for the day so that we can properly use the right type and the right amount of exercise to keep us balanced. We need to know how hot and dry we are after our day's activities if we are to workout at a level appropriate for our health.

Final Thoughts on Exercise

Currently it is popular to harken back to the olden days in order to base one's exercise regimen in the past. For example, when discussing the benefits of working toward becoming stronger at pressing weight overhead, strength coach Mark Rippetoe says:

> Working toward a bodyweight press is a laudable goal. It provides an appreciation of, and connection with, an important part of the history of weight training, a time when equipment was simple and training was straightforward. When you press, you train with Koto, Alexeyev, Starr, Grimek, and Cyr. When you press, you train much more than the shoulders and arms. You train the soul of the sport of barbell exercises.[93]

Certain ways of exercising connect us to a tradition. The desire to connect to a tradition is a very legitimate desire, seeking a foundation and a grounding for one's practice. But the tradition that Rippetoe mentions isn't even 100 years old. The real tradition is 2,500 years old and goes back to the ancient Greeks, who took exercise as seriously (and probably more seriously) than any culture in history, developing the

---

93 Rippetoe. *Strong Enough?* Wichita Falls: The Aasgaard Company, 2007. P21-2.

entire foundation of the art of exercise. If we desire a solid foundation on which to base our workout regimens, the ancient Greeks are it.

We need to keep exercise simple. All exercise is heating. Some of it is more heating than others, but it's all heating. And the heat causes dryness also, the longer one exercises, the more it dries. So it's pretty simple. Those who are hot need less exercise, just enough to strengthen and expel waste. Those who are cold need more exercise. Those who are moist need longer periods of exercise, with those who are hot needing to keep it low-level exercise. Those who are dry need short periods of exercise, with those who are cool therefore needing fairly intense forms of it.

We always take exercise, but only as much as we need. A healthy level of fitness is an easy kind of fitness. It doesn't take much. Just by grunting, panting, and sweating on a daily basis, we attain a healthy level of muscle, leanness, strength, and endurance. It's only those who demand excess that have to work hard. We can keep exercise simple if we remember that the main reasons we exercise are to ensure that we sweat, grunt, and pant enough each and every day. There's not much more to it.

Massaging for Balance

We should think of massage as a gentle form of exercise.[94] Hippocrates and Galen both considered massage to be such an integral part of exercise that it is always discussed as part of exercise itself. Hippocrates and Galen don't even make it seem like an option to not perform preparatory massage prior to a workout, and to finish a workout without massage was only a good idea under specific circumstances.[95] In general, all exercise begins and ends with massage. Massage can be taken on its own or it can be taken as both the warm-up and the cool-down to our workouts. In the previous chapter we discussed how massage is part of the warm-up and part of apotherapy, and now we'll flesh out the details.

Most importantly, massage warms the body.[96] It is heating just like other forms of exercise, but it is a very mild form of exercise, so it doesn't easily overheat the body. Massage helps to soften the body so that waste is more easily moved through the body, and it dilates one's pores, helping to expel waste through the skin. So massage is both warming and expelling, gently doing what other forms of exercise do for us.

---

94 Hygiene, p253.
95 Hygiene, p67.
96 Hygiene, p64.

When performed for a short period of time, just a few strokes of the hands, massage simply warms, reddens, and dilates the pores. When performed for a moderate amount of time, the part of the body being massaged will begin to mildly swell in response to the massage. So a moderate amount of massage moistens the body. When massage is continued for a longer period of time, the swelling will disappear and the body part will begin to shrink in response to the massage. This longer amount of massage dries the body and purges it of waste. We must therefore be careful in how long we apply massage. A little bit of massage just warms, a moderate amount moistens, and a long amount dries.

The definition of a long massage versus a short massage depends on the response of the tissues. With just a few strokes of the hands, the tissues will warm. This is a short massage. With more massage the tissues will swell. This is a moderate amount of massage. More massage will cause the tissues to contract and shrink, and that's when it is called a long massage. So it's not the amount of time but the response of the tissues that defines the length of a massage. We can't use a timer to guide us, we have to pay attention to the tissues.

The body responds to massage in the way that massage is applied. If it is applied with firm pressure, the body will harden in response. If it is applied with gentle pressure, the body will soften in response.[97] So our default amount of pressure should be a medium amount of pressure. When we encounter

97 Hygiene, p57.

an excessively hard part of the body, we should apply gentle pressure in order to help to soften it, and when we encounter an excessively soft part of the body, we should apply a firm pressure in order to harden it. We must be careful with firm pressure, of course, for it can damage the tissues if done too hard. Galen summarizes the use of pressure in massage by saying, "For if hard can contract and soft relax, those bodies which are immoderately relaxed should be rubbed hard, and those bodies which are contracted rubbed gently. And if anything is moderate, it is clear that this should be rubbed neither hard nor gently, but so far as possible avoiding either extreme."[98]

The definition of firm, medium, and gentle pressure is subjective. It is different for each person. Basically, if the pressure feels like a strong pressure, is tender, and makes one slightly tense against it, then it is firm pressure, and the tissue will harden in response. The pressure of a massage should never be so intense that one is jumping and flinching away from it, for this would be a damaging amount of pressure. A firm pressure should feel literally invigorating: it puts vigor into the tissues. If the pressure feels like a soft pressure, gentle, relaxing, and even boring, then it is gentle pressure, and the tissue will soften in response. A medium amount of pressure lies between the hard and the soft. It is a comfortable pressure that can feel slightly tender, but in general feels good.

---

98 Hygiene, p63.

So there are nine types of massage:[99] it can be applied with firm, medium, or gentle pressure, for a short, moderate, or long period of time. Each of these nine ways to apply massage have different effects on the body. The following chart should make this clear.

	Gentle Pressure	Medium Pressure	Firm Pressure
Long Duration	Softens and dries	Dries	Hardens and dries
Moderate Duration	Softens and moistens	Moistens	Hardens and moistens
Short Duration	Softens	Only warms	Hardens

When we massage the body, we must be aware of these various effects that we can have, and we must be careful to only apply massage in a balancing way. The safest form of massage is a medium pressure for a short period of time, as this will only warm the body. This should be our default way to massage unless we have a good reason to do otherwise.

Massage is the most effective tool we have for softening parts of the body that are too hard. Gentle pressure is the key to softening the body. Massage can also be used to harden parts of the body that are too soft, but this can be a very risky procedure because it requires firm pressure in the massage. Firm pressure can injure the tissues of the body if applied excessively, and for this reason we would be wise to instead

---

99 Hygiene, p66.

use exercise to harden tissues that are too soft instead of relying on massage. Galen says that massage can strengthen weak parts of the body, but it should only be applied when those weak parts are feeling healthy, and it should be avoided when a part of the body is injured.[100]

We need to understand that the ancient Greeks and Romans had slaves and servants to massage them. Few of us in today's world have the luxury of being able to afford to have someone massage us on a daily basis, so we will have to settle for self-massage. The basic technique of self-massage is to use the palms of the hands to rub the tissues of the body. We use our hands to massage the body because they are midway between soft and hard, making them the perfect structure with which to massage the body. Galen says, "... rub with the bare hands, which are midway between hard and soft, so that the body may be neither contracted and constricted nor relaxed and dilated more than is desirable, but may be kept within the bounds of nature."[101] Various positions are used to make accessing the tissues of the body easier. The details of the positions and techniques for self-massage were shown in the chapter *Exercising for Balance*. What remains is for us to discuss how to apply massage in order to prepare for exercise, for cooling-down from exercise during apotherapy, and for massage taken on its own.

Massage can be done with oil or dust, or performed dry, that is, with nothing at all. Oil is hot and moist, while dust is cold

---

100 Hygiene, p198.
101 Hygiene, p56.

and dry,[102] and dry massage is neutral. The ancients had many oils to use, but the most common was olive oil. In the cold times of the year, massaging with oil helps to keep the body warm, but in the hot times of the year, oil can cause excessive heat. Oil is extremely helpful during preparatory massage to warm the body to prepare it for exercise, especially during the cold time of the year. Oil decreases friction in massage,[103] thereby making it less forceful, and less likely to cause damage to the tissues being massaged. Dust, being cold and dry, is more appropriate in the hot times of the year to prevent excessive heating. It can be applied after exercise to cool the body, but should not be left on for too long because it will dry the body excessively. The safest bet is a dry massage, which is neutral, and therefore a more controlled way to massage. But without oil there will be more friction, and so it is easier to accidentally apply too much pressure. In general, we should massage with a little bit of oil, but for those with a hot constitution and especially during the hot times of the year, a dry massage and even a dust massage may be appropriate.

Preparatory Massage

Preparatory massage is the massage done at the start of a workout. Its purpose is to swell and redden the body, getting it ready for exercise. Preparatory massage helps to warm each part of body so that it is ready for exercise, it dilates the pores of the skin, preparing the skin to expel waste during exercise,

---

102 Hippocrates 4, Regimen 2, Ch 65.
103 Hygiene, p103.

and it encourages sweating so that waste begins to be expelled. It maximizes the benefits of exercise and minimizes the risks.[104] All forms of massage warm the body, which prepares it for the heat of exercise. And since we are preparing our bodies for vigorous exercise, we want to use a firm pressure in order to encourage the body to harden in preparation for vigorous work. But we must remember that health abhors sudden change, so we don't want to start with firm pressure. Instead, we should start with a gentle pressure and build to a firm pressure. Our purpose is not to moisten or dry the body with our preparatory massage, so we want to make it of short duration. To summarize, our preparatory massage should be a few strokes across each part of the body starting with gentle and building to firm pressure.[105] Each body part should be warm, flushed, and firm, so as to be ready for exercise.

Apotherapeutic Massage

Apotherapy is the finishing component of all exercise, designed to calm the body, prevent fatigue, and finish the beneficial effects of exercise by expelling waste and making a smooth transition from the intense heat of exercise to the mild heat of regular living. The details of apotherapy were discussed in the chapter *Exercising for Balance*, but the details of the massage component are discussed here.

Galen makes the difference between preparatory and apotherapeutic massage clear by saying: "... continuous and

104 Hygiene, p76.
105 Hygiene, p105.

vigorous massage is appropriate to preparatory exercise, but intermittent and moderate massage is appropriate to apotherapy."[106] Apotherapeutic massage is performed intermittently, spaced between various other apotherapeutic exercises. Apotherapy massage is primarily performed to expel waste and prevent fatigue, but it should also be used to balance the body. The default way to perform the massage is with a moderate pressure for a short duration, which will not harden, soften, dry, or moisten the body, instead only helping to expel waste. But if a part of the body is excessively moist, then it should be massaged for a long duration, and if a part of the body is too dry, then it should be massaged for a moderate duration. If a part of the body is too hard, then it should be performed with a gentle pressure, and if a part of the body is too soft, then it should be performed with a firm but safe pressure. Apotherapeutic massage should be balancing, but we should never lose sight of its primary purpose, which is to squeeze waste from the body so that we do not get fatigued from exercise.

Massage on its Own

Massage performed on its own can be used to help balance the body. It should be viewed as a very gentle form of exercise which heats the body and is therefore appropriate for those who are too cold. It should be performed in such a way as to balance the body, using a firm pressure on soft parts of the body, a gentle pressure on hard parts, and a moderate pressure on parts that are neither hard nor soft. It should be

---

106 Hygiene, p105.

performed for a long time on parts of the body that are too moist, for a moderate duration on parts of the body that are too dry, and for a short duration on those parts of the body that are neither too moist nor too dry. Essentially, massage on its own should be performed exactly how one performs the massage portion of apotherapy.

Galen recommends a morning massage for those who are too cold and/or fatigued, since massage will warm the body without fatiguing it much at all.[107] People who are too cold and too dry can be warmed and moistened effectively with moderate, frequent massages, perhaps on a daily basis. Those who are too hot and too moist should take infrequent, long massages, which effectively dry the body but can excessively warm a person who is already too hot.[108] A long massage can be an effective way to purge the body of waste. Those who are too moist can benefit greatly from a long massage designed to both dry the body and expel waste.

We can also take massage on its own for certain regions of the body as a therapy for parts of the body that are too cold, dry, moist, or hard. A cold part can be massaged shortly with a medium pressure. A dry region can be massaged for a moderate length of time with a medium pressure. A moist region can be massaged for a long period of time with a medium pressure. And a hard region can be massaged gently for a short period of time.

---

107 Hygiene, p137.
108 Hygiene, p200.

By making use of the information in this chapter, massage can be a highly effective tool to balance our health.

Bathing for Balance

Bathing was a common health practice in the ancient Greek and Roman worlds. Hippocrates and Galen both said that it was best done at the end of the day, after one's exercise and before one's meal.[109] One obvious reason for bathing after the activities of the day and after completing one's exercise was to clean the body of the sweat and grime of the day. It was also to refresh oneself. There is a beautiful scene in the *Odyssey* in which Odysseus bathes, washing away the exhaustion and grime of his long and perilous journey:

> Great Odysseus bathed in the river, scrubbed his body
> clean of brine that clung to his back and broad shoulders,
> scoured away the brackish scurf that caked his head.
> And then, once he had bathed all over, rubbed oil
> and donned the clothes the virgin princess gave him,
> Zeus's daughter Athena made him taller to all eyes,
> his build more massive now, and down from his brow
> she ran his curls like thick hyacinth clusters
> full of blossoms. As a master craftsman washes
> gold over beaten silver - a man the god of fire
> and Queen Athena trained in every fine technique -
> and finishes off his latest effort, handsome work,
> so she lavished splendor over his head and shoulders now.
> And down to the beach he walked and sat apart,

---

109 Food, p127.

glistening in his glory, breathtaking, yes,
and the princess gazed in wonder...[110]

Galen mentions a number of ways that ancient people cleaned themselves during their baths. Bean meal, barley meal, and washing soda (sodium carbonate) were all used to scrub the body clean.[111] So certainly bathing was about cleaning. But we must understand that ancient people had very different standards for cleanliness than we do. It was fine to only bathe a few times per month if that's what was best for one's constitution. But since it's not acceptable in our society to smell of body odor, we must bathe more frequently than Hippocrates might recommend. We need to learn to take care how we bathe and how to fit it into our daily regimen.

Obviously, submerging ourselves in water adds moisture to the body. Hippocrates says, "To refrain from baths dries, as the moisture is used up...."[112] But we can use bathing to heat, cool, moisten, soften, harden, and purge the body of waste, so there is much more to this story. Hippocrates says: "Drinkable water moistens and cools, as it gives moisture to the body. A salt bath warms and dries, as having a natural heat it draws the moisture from the body."[113] All bathing will tend to be moistening, but by adding salt, we decrease this effect. A very salty bath, such as in the ocean, can even be drying. So we can bathe in order to moisten or dry the body.

---

110 Homer. 1996. *The Odyssey*. Translated by Robert
    Fagles. New York: Penguin Group. Book 6. Lines 247-263.
111 Food, p98.
112 Hippocrates 4, Regimen 2, Ch 57, p343-5.
113 Hippocrates 4, Regimen 2, Ch 57, p343.

In addition, the temperature of the water is immensely important. A warm bath heats the body, while a cool bath cools it, and a tepid bath will neither heat nor cool the body. The following chart summarizes what we've so far discussed.

	Cool	Tepid	Warm
Heavy Salt	Cools and dries	Dries	Warms and dries
Mild Salt	Cools	Neutral	Warms
Fresh Water	Cools and moistens	Moistens	Warms and moistens

In this chapter we're going to assume the use of fresh water or lightly salted water.

The amount of time that we spend in the bath affects our balance. When talking about bathing, Hippocrates says: "First it swells, then it becomes slender...."[114] What he means is that the body takes in the moisture of the bath and swells, moistening the body, and then, after a longer period of bathing, the moisture of the body flows out, purging the body of waste. A short bath, stopped before the body swells, doesn't moisten the body much at all. A moderately long bath, stopped when the body has swollen but has not yet begun to wrinkle in response to the water, is moistening. And a long bath, only stopped when the skin of the fingers has wrinkled significantly, is purging. The following chart summarizes:

---

114 Hippocrates quoted in Hygiene, p75.

	Cool	Tepid	Warm
Long Duration	Cools, moistens, purges	Moistens, purges	Heats, moistens, purges
Moderate Duration	Cools, moistens	Moistens	Heat, moistens
Short Duration	Cools	Neutral	Heats

Purging the body of excrement is one of the great benefits of bathing and this only occurs with long bathing. Long baths can be used when other forms of expelling excrement are not balancing or have failed to fully expel waste. For example, if it's too hot and dry to expel one's waste by lots of exercise and long massage (which are both heating and drying), then a long cool bath can be very helpful to expel waste, for it can be cooling and moistening in the process.

If relaxing while bathing is one of the aims, then a cup for pouring the bath water over one's body is very useful. There are few things more relaxing than comfortable water poured over the skin. It's much like a massage, and it takes almost no effort. It's hypnotic.

So far we've discussed cool, tepid, and warm baths, all of which we'll define as comfortable baths because all three of these temperatures feel comfortable to the bather. There is another category of bathing which makes use of either uncomfortably hot or uncomfortably cold water. These are not painfully hot or painfully cold temperatures, which would be imbalancing and potentially injurious temperatures to use, but these are temperatures that are not relaxing or calming to the bather. In fact, these are temperatures that make us more tense, for we tense against the water. Uncomfortable baths therefore cause a hardening of the tissues of the body, while comfortable bathing, being relaxing, causes a softening of the body's tissues. The pores of the body close when in uncomfortable water, and so there is little flow of moisture into the body and little flow of excrement out of the body when bathing in uncomfortable water. For this reason, moderate and long uncomfortable baths do not moisten or purge the body, and short baths of this sort do not moisten. We will call these uncomfortable baths hot and cold to distinguish them from their comfortable counterparts: warm and cool. The effects of all five temperatures can be seen in the following chart.

	Cold	Cool	Tepid	Warm	Hot
Long Duration	Chills*, hardens	Cools, moistens softens, purges	Softens, moistens, purges	Warms, moistens, softens, purges	Heats*, hardens
Mod. Duration	Chills*, hardens	Cools, softens, moistens	Softens, moistens	Warms, softens, moistens	Heats*, hardens
Short Duration	Cools, hardens	Cools, softens	Softens	Warms, softens	Warms, hardens

* A moderate or a long stay in uncomfortably hot or cold water is rarely a balancing activity and could easily cause severe imbalances. They are not recommended.

The effects of a short dip in cold water is commended by Galen, who says: "[People] are hungrier than usual, after cold bathing, and digest better, and are less thirsty."[115] Cold water strengthens the whole body and makes the skin tough. It's best to exercise and then get into the cold all at once to avoid shivering. It can progress to icy cold, but not at first. Get out and rub with oil until the body is warm. Then eat more food than usual, but drink less. A second dip in the cold after the oiling is often very useful. The length of time in the cold should be as long as possible that still allows the color of the skin and the warmth of the body to return very quickly after exiting the bath and massaging with oil. This is how Galen suggests we take cold baths.

Since even a moderately long, moderately warm bath can cause excessive moistening and softening of the body, we must be careful how we bathe. Hot and moist people need to make sure that bathing does not cause them to become excessively moist. So they need to take short baths certainly, ideally cool. Cold baths will constrict the skin and prevent moisture from coming in, so these will help to both cool the body and prevent excessive moisture. But of course, moist people need help expelling waste, and constricting the skin to prevent the influx of moisture also prevents the expulsion of waste. So when waste is excessive, a longer tepid bath may be in order, always noting that this will increase moisture. A long hot bath is rarely a balancing idea for these people. Hot and moist people should consider short, cold bathing their ideal, with short cool baths being another good option. Adding

---

115 Hygiene, p112.

salt to the bath will help prevent the bath from adding excessive moisture.

Hot and dry people need moisture, so long baths are appropriate for them. But these baths should not be hot or even warm. Tepid or cool baths are most appropriate. And these baths should not be cold or hot because that would close the skin, preventing the moisture of the bath from being absorbed into the body. Cool or tepid, moderately long baths are their ideal.

Cold and dry people need baths the most. Long, warm baths are very beneficial, adding moisture and warmth to the body. But it's important that these baths not be too hot, which would close the skin from absorbing the moisture. These people should avoid cold bathing. Moderately long warm baths are best for them.

Cold and moist people can benefit from warm bathing, but these baths must be short to avoid excessive moisture, and hot water can be helpful to close the skin and prevent excessive moisture from accumulating. In the same way that hot and moist people need help expelling waste, cold and moist people do also, so long baths are occasionally appropriate. Adding salt helps to keep baths from being too imbalancing for these people.

We have not yet mentioned showers in this discussion of bathing, and that's because Hippocrates and Galen do not mention them. In the ancient world, it was common practice to bathe, not shower. Some obvious things can be said about showers, however. For one thing, showers do not immerse the body in water, and so are much less moistening than are baths. But the heat or cold of a shower will still have its effect, and so will the comfort or discomfort, albeit less so. The key difference between showers and bathing is that in a bathe one is covered, and stays covered, by the water. In a shower, one can go in and out of the water with ease. An uncomfortably hot or cold bath is a continuously uncomfortable event, while an uncomfortable shower can be intermittently uncomfortable. In addition, one reclines and rests in a bath, while one stands in a shower. A bath is therefore naturally more relaxing, and therefore softening to the body, while a shower is less relaxing and therefore less softening.

Showers can be understood as a faster, easier way to clean oneself, and as a less powerful form of bathing. In our modern world, in which we cannot be dirty and smelly without suffering social ostracization, showers make a lot of sense for those who need to clean themselves but who need to avoid the strong effects of bathing. In particular, those who are too moist should consider showers as part of their regular regimen. On the other hand, those who are too dry should strongly consider making bathing instead of showering their common practice.

Bathing is a powerful tool for balancing the body and it is therefore also a dangerous one. Even a moderately long, moderately warm bath can severely imbalance a person who is already too hot and too moist. Remember, Hippocrates sometimes told moist people to bathe only a few times per month. It might be best for these people to bathe only a few times per month and only take short showers on the other days.

With bathing, even moderation may not be safe. The benefits of bathing are immense. It can be used to heat, cool, moisten, dry (with lots of salt), relax, soften, harden, and expel waste without exercising or drying the body. No other tool at our disposal offers us so many options for helping to balance ourselves, and conversely no other tool can imbalance us so insidiously if used inappropriately.

Eating for Balance

"[The power of food] is probably the most important of all medical subjects." - Galen[116]

The ancient way of imagining things is that the activity of life melts the flesh of our bodies, and it is only by eating food that we nourish ourselves back to health. Food replenishes what we lose each day: "By food, therefore, we replace whatever solid substance has escaped, and by drink we replenish the liquid, thus restoring both to their original proportion."[117] So eating is first and foremost about replenishing the body. Our meals must be appropriately nourishing to the depletion of the day, a hard day of manual labor or exercise replenished with thicker, nourishing foods, and a light day of rest replenished with a thinner, less nourishing meal.

But the digestion and assimilation of food isn't perfect: "... since the substance of foods is not all nutritious, and on this account the surplus of it remains as something deleterious...."[118] Some types of food are more easily assimilated into the body, such as lettuce, while other foods are not as easily assimilated, such as beef. The difficulties of digestion and assimilation lead to waste material and

---

116 Food, p68.
117 Hygiene, p7-8.
118 Hygiene, p235.

excrement, which we must eliminate from our bodies through urine, feces, sweat, and the breath. If this process were perfect, we would remain in perfect health and never grow old: "For if there were no failure, either in replacing the wastes or in the excrements remaining within, the animal would be healthy and would flourish for a long time."[119] Unfortunately, this process is not perfect, but the more perfect we make it, the healthier we will remain and the longer we will live.

All foods are imperfect and therefore contain some form of negative power on the body. Some foods make our flesh soft and spongy. Other foods make our flesh hard. Some foods thicken the blood, clogging the function of the body and leading to imbalances, while other foods excessively thin the blood.[120] What we want is to be balanced, and to be balanced we need balanced blood. Galen defines this balanced state of blood by saying: "What I mean by average is blood which is not too thin and watery, yet not particularly thick."[121] When blood gets imbalanced, it becomes attractive to insects, in particular to fleas.[122] Blood that is too thick makes us excessively cold and dry, while blood that is too thin makes us excessively hot and moist.[123]

So the foods that we eat must combine to make a meal that is nourishing enough to replenish us and able to be digested and assimilated without significant problems. The trouble is

---

119 Hygiene, p10.
120 Food, p116.
121 Food, p178.
122 Food, p116.
123 Food, p97.

that foods that are nourishing are also thick. Thick foods are hard to digest and can thicken the blood excessively. Beef is a good example of a thick food. On the other hand, thin foods, such as lettuce, offer us very little nourishment. Someone who ate nothing but beef would certainly be nourished, but would suffer from poor digestion and thick blood. And someone who ate only lettuce would never get enough nourishment, but would be able to digest and assimilate his or her food quite well. We must be clear about the ancient idea of nourishment. Foods were called nourishing if they replenished the body in a relatively small bulk. For example, beef is more nourishing than lettuce because one can eat a much smaller amount of beef to replenish the body compared to how much lettuce one would need to eat in order to replenish the body. If we take the modern notion of calories, the idea becomes clear. Essentially, nourishing foods are high in calories.

Thick nourishment is harder to digest, is digested slowly, and replenishes us more, while thin nourishment is easier to digest, is digested quickly, and replenishes us less.[124] The key is to combine thick and thin foods. The thick food provides nourishment while the thin food eases the process of digesting and assimilating the thick food, resulting in more balanced blood. Combining beef and lettuce is a more balancing way to eat than having either one by itself. Lettuce alone would thin our blood and beef alone would thicken it.

---

124 Food, p101, p110-11, p155.

So we need to combine thick foods and thin foods. But if thin foods, which digest quickly, are eaten after thick foods, which digest slowly and therefore sit in the bowels like a heavy glob, then the thin foods will begin to rot and cause indigestion. Galen explains: "... [thin foods] rot as they rest on top. It is essential to bear in mind these basic facts which are applicable to [all thin foods that pass quickly: they] must be eaten before other foods, for then they pass through the body quickly, and lead the way for other foods."[125] Whenever we don't digest our food well, we get the uncomfortable feeling of something like clay sitting in our bowels that causes flatulent bloating, headache, and blurred vision.[126] Thin foods eaten after thick foods make the meal rot and therefore cause bad digestion, and thick foods eaten without preparation by thin foods create a large lump that is very hard to digest. So thin foods must have a clear passage through the intestines, and therefore thin foods must be eaten before thick foods. This is all well and good, since the thin foods prepare the stomach, intestines, and liver for the coming thick foods, helping the thick foods to be better digested. The thin foods can act as a signal to the body to prepare for more food. If we don't prepare the stomach with thin foods and jump straight to eating thick foods, then the thick foods will sit in our bowels like large thick clumps which constrict our stomachs, causing a feeling of heaviness and cramping, making breathing difficult, and even causing fainting and cold sweats.[127] So an ideal meal will combine thick and thin foods to offer a properly

---

125 Food, p124-5.
126 Food, p85.
127 Food, p151.

nourishing meal that creates balanced blood and that is digested well because the thin foods precede and prepare the body for the thick foods. We should not only combine beef and lettuce, but have the lettuce first in order to prepare for the beef.

In general, thick foods are animal products, grains, beans, and seeds, and thin foods are fruits and vegetables. There are of course various degrees of thickness and thinness in foods. Beef is one of the thickest foods we can eat, whereas fish is only mildly thickening. Garlic is as thin as any food can be, and lettuce only mildly thinning. So the very thin garlic can prepare and thin in a more balancing way for the very thickening beef, and the less thinning lettuce balances better with the less thickening fish.

Eating is first and foremost about replenishing the body. Those who are highly active, such as athletes in training, need more nourishment and so thicker foods, while sedentary and ill people need less nourishment and thinner foods. Galen says that athletes would be unhealthy on a diet of mostly vegetables, and sedentary people would be unhealthy on a diet of mostly meat. Heavy athletes eat pork and heavy bread that is not easily spoiled and hard to disperse, allowing them to exercise hard all day, but a normal person would be ill very fast with this kind of food, as an athlete would be very hurt living off vegetables and barley juice.[128] So an active athlete would want to skew the balance toward the thick side by pairing the less thinning lettuce with the very thickening

---

128 Food, p81.

beef, while the sedentary person would want to skew to the thin by pairing the very thinning garlic with the less thickening fish.

Balance

But food is not only about replenishing ourselves, for all foods also carry the power to shove us around on the wobble board of health. Some foods are heating, while others are cooling. Some foods are drying, and others moistening. Wheat is hot and dry, for example, while barley is cold and moist. Wheat is therefore much more appropriate during the cold and moist times of the year and for those with a cold and moist constitution, while the cold and moist barley is a more balancing choice during the hot and dry times of the year and for people with a hot and dry constitution.

All foods have at least some degree of power to either heat, cool, dry, or moisten,[129] and from the mixing of each food's unique powers comes its flavor:[130] bitter, sour, sweet, or salty. Some foods are close to flavorless, but all foods have some flavor, and it is the flavor that tells us their power. In order for us to understand the power of foods to heat, cool, dry, and moisten, we must learn about the power of flavors.

First we must compare and contrast the powers of the bitter and the sour flavors. The bitter flavor is heating and drying.[131]

---

129 Food, p72.
130 Food, p76.
131 Food, p123.

It expels moisture from the body.[132] Bitter foods cut through thick juices and help to thin them, making them easier to digest.[133] Bitter foods are powerful in their heating and drying effect. Their power is very helpful for those who are cold and moist, but for those who are hot and dry they can be dangerous. Galen warns us to "... avoid continual use of all bitter foods, especially when the person eating them is by nature rather [hot and dry]. For such foods are suitable only for those who [are excessively cold and moist]."[134] Galen is here referring to such powerfully bitter foods as garlic and onions, but the same is applicable to all foods that are bitter, just to a lesser degree. This includes coffee and tea.

The sour flavor is very different than the bitter flavor, for it is cooling instead of heating. While bitter foods open, expand, and heat, sour foods close, contract, and cool.[135] Sour foods thicken the moisture in the body and the food in the bowels by sucking the moisture out of the body, so sour foods are also drying.[136] This thickening effect slows the digestion,[137] and this can be very strengthening for the stomach, helping to keep it functioning well.[138] The sour flavor stimulates the appetite, making sour foods good appetizers.[139]

---

132 Hygiene, p43.
133 Food, p75.
134 Food, p153.
135 Food, p77.
136 Hygiene, p43.
137 Food, p96-8.
138 Food, p65.
139 Hippocrates 4, Regimen 2, Ch 56.

Although most sour foods are thin foods, by being sour they carry the power to thicken, and so sour foods are appropriate to eat at the end of meals. The sour flavor thickens the end of the meal, ensuring that things are digested smoothly by ensuring the final foods of the meal are made very thick so as to prevent them from rotting and causing indigestion. Eating what is sour before what is moist, fat, and sweet can cause stoppage of the stomach,[140] so we must always emphasize the sour flavor at the end of a meal, not at the start.

Both bitter and sour foods are therefore good for the digestion as long as they are used at appropriate times in the meal. Bitter foods thin our food and so help the digestion at the start of a meal, while sour foods thicken our food and are therefore helpful at the end of a meal. If bitter foods were eaten at the end of a meal, then the end of the meal would be thinned and rot too easily. And if sour foods were eaten at the start of the meal, then the start of the meal would be thickened and clog the rest of the meal. It's important to understand that it is the strength of the flavor that matters for these effects. Taking a little bit of sour vinegar on a salad to start the meal isn't going to clog one's digestion, but eating a sour apple could very well do so. Likewise, seasoning your meat with garlic at the end of the meal isn't going to rot the meal, but eating three cloves of raw garlic most certainly will. The sour flavor can whet the appetite, so it can be used at the start of the meal as long as the sour flavor isn't prominent and overpowering.

---

140 Hygiene, p42.

As opposed as the flavors of bitter and sour are to one another, they both share three common things. First, they are both drying. Both bitter and sour foods make the overall meal a drier meal. This is balancing for those who are too moist, and imbalancing for those who are too dry. Second, excess amounts of either bitter or sour foods can stop the stomach from functioning and severely inhibit digestion,[141] so it's important to not overdo either of these flavors. A single food, course, or meal should never heavily emphasize either the bitter or sour flavors. A stomach that is too dry from an excessive amount of bitter or sour foods simply cannot digest food. Eating raw radishes by themselves, for example, is just too bitter for most stomachs to tolerate, and drinking straight lemon juice is just too sour.

The third commonality between bitter and sour flavors is that they both offer very little nourishment to the body.[142] Most foods that are bitter or sour are thin foods, offering little nourishment. It is the relatively flavorless and especially the sweet foods that nourish the body. Galen tells us that "... whatever is sour and bitter furnishes little nutrition to the body, whilst whatever is flavorless, and even more so whatever is sweet, provides a lot of nourishment."[143]

Relatively flavorless foods are those that do not have a pronounced flavor, being only slightly bitter, sour, sweet, or salty. A good example of this can be seen by comparing garlic to carrots. Both garlic and carrots have a bitter flavor,

141 Hygiene, p42.
142 Food, p149.
143 Food, p149.

but the garlic is much stronger than the carrot in this way. Carrots are relatively flavorless compared to garlic, and are therefore more nourishing and less heating and drying than garlic. It is the sweet flavor that signals the most nourishing of foods.[144] If one eats two different apples, one sweeter than the other, it is the sweeter apple that provides more nourishment.

The sweet flavor, like the bitter flavor, is heating.[145] But unlike both bitter foods and sour foods, sweet foods are moistening. So sweet foods are more appropriate for those who are cold and dry and during the cold and dry times of the year. Sweet foods in general are harmful to inflammations of the liver and spleen[146] because their hot moisture can be sticky and clog the flow between these organs and the digestive track, causing indigestion and causing the blood to become imbalanced. We must be careful that our meals are not too sweet, which is a very common problem. Most of us overemphasize the sweet flavor in our meals.

The salty flavor, like the bitter flavor, stimulates the bowels and speeds digestion. Salty sauces help to keep the bowels moving and are appropriate at the beginning of meals. Salt is also drying.

The four flavors each have a combined power to heat, cool, dry, and/or moisten, and these powers can be either balancing or imbalancing. We must take into consideration

---

144 Food, p149. Hippocrates 4, Regimen 2, Ch 56.
145 Hippocrates 4, Regimen 2, Ch 56.
146 Food, p116.

the replenishment of our body through nourishment, the thickness and thinness of the foods, and the heating, cooling, drying, and moistening effects of those foods. Galen summarizes nicely:

> For if the human body should really be average in temperament, it should be kept in its present state by nourishment that is of average temperament. If, on the other hand, it should be cooler, hotter, drier or wetter, it would be wrong to serve food and drink that was average in temperament, because it is necessary for each of these bodies to be shifted in the opposite direction by as much as they depart from the genuinely median state. This will be by means of whatever is the opposite to the existing bad temperament.[147]

So our food must nourish us appropriately and keep us balanced.

Just as thick and thin foods must be combined in a meal in order to help to keep the blood from becoming too thick or too thin, we must combine flavors in our meals in order to balance the heating, cooling, drying, and moistening effects of foods. Barley, being cold and moist, mixes well with hot and dry things such as lentils and beets. Barley alone will cool and moisten, while lentils alone will heat and dry, but mixed together they are well-balanced.

Cooking and Seasoning Food

Fortunately we can control our meals by how we prepare our foods. The way a food is cooked and seasoned can

---

147 Food, p74.

remarkably change its effect. How we cook our foods alters them: "... nothing that has been cooked can really retain its own juice; instead it loses everything if it has been cooked for a long time."[148] So cooking is a great tool to help to balance the effects of food.

We can make food more moistening and thinner by boiling it.[149] On the other hand, we can make food drier and thicker by roasting it or frying it.[150] Foods grilled and roasted are thicker and drier than raw because the fire has taken away the moisture, the juice, and the fat.[151] And if we want to cook our food without dramatically changing its power, we can bake it. Galen summarizes: "Everything that is eaten after roasting or frying furnishes the body with a drier food, whilst everything boiled beforehand in water provides a moister food, whereas everything seasoned in a casserole falls between these."[152] So there is a spectrum for how cooking affects our food. Roasting and frying is the most drying and thickening, then comes baking which has a fairly neutral effect on the food, and then comes steaming which moistens and thins the food, followed by boiling which has the most moistening and thinning effect.

---

148 Food, p141.
149 Food, p71.
150 Food, p100.
151 Hippocrates 4, Regimen 2, Ch 56.
152 Food, p155.

	Thick/Thin	Dry/Moist
Roast/Fry	Very thickening	Very drying
Bake	Mildly thickening	Mildly drying
Steam	Mildly thinning	Mildly moistening
Boil	Very thinning	Very moistening

The effect of boiling can be fine-tuned:

> There is also a considerable difference in the method of seasoning. Whatever is full of wine and [salty water] is drier than when they are omitted; whatever lacks these, but contains either a lot of new wine boiled down, which some people name reduced wine, or is boiled in what is called simple, plain and white sauce, is far moister than what has been mentioned before. But everything cooked only in water is even moister than these.[153]

All boiling makes food moister and thinner, but boiling in wine or salt water is less moistening and less thinning. Cooking foods in oil makes them hotter.[154] Fat is heating, and so adding oil makes the food more heating.

In fact, how we season our food has the greatest effect on our food:

> The greatest difference in preparation lies in the power of whatever is added to them, since these are all drying, although some more, others less so. They include the seeds of dill, celery, caraway, bastard lovage, cumin and some other seeds like them, whilst of the plants they include leeks,

153 Food, p155. Hippocrates 4, Regimen 2, Ch 56.
154 Hippocrates 4, Regimen 2, Ch 56.

onions, dill, thyme, savory, pennyroyal, sweet mint, marjoram and everything else belonging to the business of cooking....[155]

The following table summarizes:

Light Seasoning	Moderate Seasoning	Heavy Seasoning
Barely drying	Drying	Very drying

So we can make a course drier and thicker by seasoning it heavily, and by baking it, and even more so by roasting or frying it. If we want our course to be moister and thinner, then we can only lightly season it so that the seasonings don't dry and thicken it much, and we can steam it or make it even moister and thinner by boiling it. If we boil with water then we will really moisten and thin the food, and we can lessen this by boiling in salt water, and we can lessen it even more by boiling in wine. If we are trying to make a fairly balanced meal, then we should avoid the extremes: that of roasting or frying with heavy seasoning, and that of boiling in water with light seasoning. Instead, if we roast or fry then we should only lightly season, if we bake we may season a bit more, if we steam we should season even more, and if we boil then it should be in salty water or wine and should be seasoned well. These combinations allow us to cook in any way that seems appetizing while balancing the effect of the cooking with the effect of the seasoning to make a fairly well-balanced course.

---

155 Food, p157.

	Light Seasoning	Moderate Seasoning	Heavy Seasoning
Roast/Fry	Balancing		
Bake		Balancing	
Steam		Balancing	
Boil in Wine or Salt		Balancing	
Boil in Water			Balancing

So the way that we cook and season our food is very important. In general, food should be prepared to be balanced. Hippocrates summarizes how foods should be prepared: "Take away their power from strong foods by boiling and cooling many times; remove moisture from moist things by grilling and roasting them; soak and moisten dry things, soak and boil salt things, bitter and sharp things mix with sweet, and astringent things mix with oily."[156] It is the strong properties of foods that harm us, the strong heating effect of garlic for example, or the excessive sweetness of sugar. If we prepare various foods so as to calm their effects, combine them with other foods that help to neutralize their effects, and order them appropriately in a meal, then we can make eating a very balancing activity.

---

156 Hippocrates 4, Regimen 2, Ch 56.

Meals

This all brings us to the concept of meals. It is the combination of foods into a meal that allows us to replenish ourselves in a balancing way. Meals should progress from thin foods to thick foods, providing a balanced nourishment that keeps our blood from becoming too thick or too thin, and that keeps our digestion and assimilation working as perfectly as possible. Meals should also combine foods so that there is an overall balancing effect from the powers of the foods, making the meal as a whole not too hot, cold, moist, or dry.

The power of thick foods is primarily in their ability to offer enough nourishment that we can replenish ourselves, and the power of thin foods is in their ability to balance the effects of the thick foods so that our meal is digestible and balancing. "[Most foods] generally have something in common with the extremes, whilst some acquire a central position through two things of equal power being blended...."[157] Combining cool and moist barley with hot and dry lentils is a good example. If we mix food appropriately, we can be nourished and balanced by our meals.

Ancient meals included many courses. In imagining an ancient meal, it is important to know that each course was accompanied by bread.[158] They started with appetizers to help to stimulate the appetite and to help prepare the

---

157 Food, p98.
158 Smith. *The Frugal Gourmet Cooks Three Ancient Cuisines*. New York: William Morrow and Company, Inc, 1989. P65.

digestion for the meal. Appetizers are thin foods that are laxative and digestive and stimulating for the appetite. Then they ate vegetables, which would pass quickly and help to balance the meal by adding thin nourishment. Then they ate the thicker and harder food, such as meat. And then they finished with what Galen called 'side dishes,' which were small dishes of tasty food eaten primarily for pleasure. These 'side dishes' were the hardest to digest and saved for the end of the meal so as not to interfere with the rest of the meal's digestion.[159] Usually they saved most of their drinking for during the meal, drinking between courses, and especially at the end of the meal. It was during the drinking at the end of the meal that the 'side dishes' were served. This can be thought of as the equivalents of today's dessert course, but these 'side dishes' could also be savory and deep fried foods.

The ancients ate one and sometimes two meals per day. This can be understood from the following comment by Hippocrates: "For the great majority of men can follow indifferently either the one habit or the other, and can take lunch or only one daily meal,"[160] and from Galen: "... to eat once instead of twice, or instead of once, to eat twice or even more frequently."[161] The ancient discussion about how many meals a person should have in a day focused on the options of one meal or two. This is a far cry from the popular trends of today which recommend up to six meals per day. Hippocrates summarizes the findings of the ancients on this matter:

---

159 Food, p107.
160 Hippocrates 1, Ancient Medicine, Ch 10.
161 Hygiene, p45.

"Taking one meal a day reduces, dries and binds the bowels, because, through the warmth of the soul the moisture is consumed from out of the belly and the flesh. To take lunch has effects opposite to those of taking one meal only."[162] So having one meal per day is drying,[163] thinning, and potentially constipating, while having two meals per day is moistening, thickening, and loosening to the bowels. Those who are too moist and during the moist times of the year should probably settle on one meal per day, while those who are too dry and during the dry times of the year should probably eat an additional meal per day.

We must ensure that we eat enough food, for if we allow ourselves to become undernourished, there are just as severe of problems as if we were to become over-nourished. Hippocrates says, "But as it is, if a man take insufficient food, the mistake is as great as that of excess, and harms the man just as much. For abstinence has upon the human constitution a most powerful effect, to enervate, to weaken and to kill. Depletion produces many other evils, different from those of repletion, but just as severe."[164] So perhaps the most important reason that one would choose to have more than one meal per day is that eating an excessive amount of food at any one time can cause stoppage of the stomach[165] and thus severely disturb digestion. So our meals cannot be huge. Our meals can be large and satisfying, but not excessively

---

162 Hippocrates 4, Regimen 2, Ch 60.
163 Hippocrates 4, Aphorisms, Book 7, Ch 60.
164 Hippocrates 1, Ancient Medicine, Ch 9.
165 Hygiene, p42.

huge so as to cause indigestion. So if we need more food, then we should simply have an additional meal, perhaps even a third meal during the day, but this is only of use to those who are very active and so need a lot of nourishment which simply cannot be met by one meal alone.

Galen makes the case for a balanced approach to meals. Even those who desperately need to eat less food should not stop eating entirely, "... for to give more to those needing evacuation is wholly inappropriate, and on the other hand not to feed them at all is unsafe, and injurious to the stomach, and impairs its strength, and increases indigestion."[166] It's important that we eat enough but not too much food, and this is best accomplished with one or two satisfying meals per day.

But although Hippocrates may prescribe eating only one or two meals per day, we must remember that health abhors sudden change. People suffer greatly when they suddenly skip a meal that they are accustomed to taking, or when they eat a meal that they do not normally take.[167] Usually ancient people ate one main meal at the end of the day, and sometimes had a small meal near the start of the day. The one or two meals per day regimen should be an eventual ideal for most of us, but a sudden change in diet creates problems. So if one who normally eats five meals per day tries to suddenly change to eating one meal per day, he or she will almost certainly become ill. It would be better to just

---

166 Hygiene, p157-8.
167 Hippocrates 1, Ancient Medicine, Ch 10.

emphasize one meal, and slowly start to shrink and then eliminate the other four meals.

Drink

Drinking is an important part of every meal. Culpeper, a physician from the 1600s who carried on the tradition of Galen and Hippocrates, gives us some great advice about drinking, saying:

> 1) Accustom your body to drink as little as may be between meals, 2) drink not at all at meals before you have eaten something, 3) drink the smallest [weakest] beer first, and the strongest afterward... and 4) drink often at meals whether you be [thirsty] or not, for it: 1) helps digestion, 2) mingles the meat in the stomach, and 3) helps it to pass....[168]

So drinking is not only important during a meal, it should ideally be saved for meals, with only occasional sips as needed during the rest of the day. Liquids should be imagined as food. Hippocrates says: "Strong drink dispels hunger."[169] Liquids are part of our meals.

Thin liquids, the most thin being water, should precede thicker liquids, such as alcohol. The stronger the alcohol, the thicker it is. A light white wine is therefore thinner than a heavy red wine. So our meals could progress from water to light white wine to strong red wine.

------

168 Culpeper's commentary on Art. Ch 85.
169 Hippocrates 4, Aphorisms, Ch 2.21.

The temperature of liquids is important. Cold water can cool a stomach that is too hot.[170] But we must bear in mind that very cold liquids (such as ice water) thicken whatever is in the bowels, which can cause serious indigestion, and very hot liquids (the way that many of us take our coffee or tea) can do likewise by heating and thereby drying what is in the bowels.[171] We are much safer to take our liquids at comfortable temperatures. Bear in mind that Hippocrates here is talking of "excessive cold," and "excess of heat." Uncomfortably cold or hot drinks are not wise parts of our meals, but comfortably warm and cool drinks are fine.

Planning a Meal

When planning a meal, it is best to first choose the thick nourishment, for this is the food that will replenish us. We need to ensure that we get enough but not too much of this thick nourishment. All meat, poultry, fish, eggs, milk, beans, and grains are thick nourishment. Once we've chosen our thick food, we should then decide how to prepare it, often preparing it in such a way as to balance its strong powers. If we're having beef, then we may want to roast it in order to dry this moist food. Or we may want to combine two thick foods in order to balance them out, such as mixing barley and lentils, the barley being cold and moist and the lentils being hot and dry, combining into a fairly neutral course.

After choosing our thick nourishment and how we will prepare it for the meal, we should choose our thin nourishment. This

---

170 Food, p166.
171 Hippocrates 4, Regimen 2, Ch 60.

food should balance the power of our thick nourishment both by thinning the overall effect of the meal to an appropriate amount (thinning it a lot if we are sedentary, and thinning it not much at all if we are very active) and by balancing the heating, cooling, drying, and moistening effect of the thick nourishment so as to balance us overall. If we're having a relatively hot and dry thick nourishment such as fish, then we'll probably want to have a relatively cool and moist thin nourishment such as lettuce in order to ensure that the meal doesn't imbalance us. If we're having a relatively cool and moist thick nourishment such as barley, then we'll probably want to have a relatively hot and dry thin nourishment such as beets.

Of course, if we are imbalanced in any direction, being too hot, too cold, too dry, or too moist, then we will want to slightly adjust our meal in order to adjust a bit in the opposite direction. This must always be accomplished with subtlety because health abhors sudden changes, and strong flavors and foods can easily upset our digestion and balance. So if we're too cold and moist, then we'd want to add a serving of cabbage, for example, to our meal, not have five servings of cabbage seasoned heavily with garlic, onions, and cayenne pepper, which would be severely heating and drying.

In all of this it's important to think of taste and pleasure: "Indeed, I do not consider it right for a doctor to be completely ignorant of the art of cooking, because whatever tastes good is easier to digest than other dishes which may be equally as healthy."[172] Boiling beef may be a way of making it thinner and therefore potentially more balancing, but it is also not a very elegant or particularly appetizing way to eat beef. One hopes that a piece of filet mignon never finds itself boiled in a pot of water! Knowing this, when we are going to have a meal of something like beef cooked to taste, it will be a strong and potentially imbalancing part of the meal, and so we should prepare for this by ensuring that the rest of the meal helps to balance the potential imbalance. Seasoned and roasted beef, for example, is a thicker form of an already thick food. The thin part of our meal should be very thin in order to help balance this tasty dish of beef.

It is best to choose at least one thin food to start as an appetizer. This should be a very thin, quickly passing, and easily digestible food that whets the appetite and prepares the digestive tract for thicker food. Radishes, olives, cucumbers, melons, and mulberries all fit well as appetizers. The thin foods can be imagined as appetizing medicines that are taken prior to the real nourishment of the thick foods. These medicines prepare our appetite and digestion, balance the soon to come thick foods, and balance our overall health on the wobble board.

After selecting our thick and thin foods for the meal, it is time to choose a sour food to end the meal. The sour flavor contracts and squeezes the bowels, helping to signal the end of the meal, and helping to move the meal along down the digestive tract. Apples are a great choice for this part of the

---

172 Food, p131.

meal. All apples, even those that are bitter or sweet, have a sour flavor also, and so the sour flavor does a good job of finishing the meal. Various apples can be bitter, sweet, or quite sour, and apples can be eaten raw or cooked in various ways, allowing us a great amount of flexibility in how this finish to the meal can affect us.

After the meal proper is completed with a sour course, we are left to drinking and to eating small amounts of foods eaten only for pleasure. These foods can be extremely hard to digest because they will sit at the end of an entire meal's worth of food, and so won't interfere with our digestion much at all. It is at this time that hard to digest foods such as cheese, candy, fried foods, and complicated desserts should be eaten. These foods are eaten slowly, relished for their pleasure, and not taken in excessive amounts.

Once we have the foods that we will be eating for our meal, we can select our drinks. Between each course we should drink some liquid, more if we are thirsty and/or dry, and less if we aren't thirsty or if we are excessively moist. The drinks for the meal should progress from the thinnest to the thickest of drinks, with water being the obvious starter, and harder alcohols coming at the end of the meal. One example is to have water after the thin foods, a mild white wine after the thick foods, and a strong red wine after the meal.

Thick Nourishment

Most of the nourishment of a meal will come from the thick nourishment of meats, poultry, fish, eggs, dairy foods, beans, and grains. These foods provide lots of nourishment and allow us to replenish ourselves.

Meat, poultry, and fish are the prime examples of thick nourishment. They are highly nourishing and provide thick and hard nourishment. All animal flesh is heating, but not all animal flesh is the same. Some flesh, such as beef, is extremely thick and hard to digest, while some flesh, such as soft fish, is relatively thin and easy to digest. Hard flesh is harder to digest and makes thicker juices than soft flesh.[173] In general, meat is the thickest and hardest of the types of animal flesh, while fish is the thinnest and softest. Poultry lies in the middle of this spectrum, and is oftentimes the most balancing choice. Poultry is less nourishing but easier to digest than meat[174] but more nourishing and harder to digest than fish. In fact, poultry is one of the few foods that easily converts into balanced flesh and blood of the human body, and therefore should be the default choice for most people.

Meats, such as beef, pork, and lamb, offer a thicker and harder nourishment than poultry. They are harder to digest and make thicker blood.[175] They are appropriate for those with thinned blood, which is most likely to occur in those who are very active, such as athletes in training. Pork is the most nourishing of the meats and the most easily converted into the flesh of the body. Galen says, "Of all foods... pork is the most nutritious. ... Athletes display the most striking proof of this fact, for if one day they eat an equal weight of some other

173 Food, p182.
174 Food, p170.
175 Food, p154.

food when training for their exercises, on the next day they grow weaker... [and show] signs of malnutrition."[176] Beef is drier than pork[177] and can cause excessively thick blood.[178]

Fish offers a thinner and softer nourishment than poultry, and is therefore easier to digest. It makes a thinner blood, and so is appropriate for those whose blood is too thick due to a sedentary lifestyle or illness. The harder the flesh of the fish, the thicker is its nourishment, and therefore some of the harder fish offer a nourishment that is basically equivalent to the very balanced nourishment of poultry. Fish that live in deep, windy oceans along the rocks are the best type of fish for us to eat, for their flesh is harder and therefore more easily converted into our bodies.[179] Fish flesh should be flavorful, pleasant, and without oiliness. Fish such as tilapia are suitable to human nature and can be eaten often.[180] Tilapia is soft and friable, while salmon is oily and hard and so needs marjoram, mustard, and vinegar to be more digestible.[181] Tuna has a particularly hard flesh.[182]

Other common seafood comes closer to meat than to fish. Crabs, lobster, and shrimp/prawns have hard flesh and so are hard to digest but nutritious.[183]

---

176 Food, p154.
177 Food, p155.
178 Food, p154.
179 Food, p178.
180 Food, p177.
181 Food.
182 Food, p186.
183 Food, p185.

Hippocrates says: "All birds are drier than beasts. ... [and] to the flesh of fish, these are the driest."[184] So meats are the moistest, fish the driest, and poultry is in the middle of these extremes, which again makes poultry the balanced choice. The following table summarizes the powers of animal flesh:

Fish	Mildly hot and moist	Mildly thick
Poultry	Hot and moist	Thick
Meat	Very hot and moist	Very thick

Fat is itself heating, moistening, and filling.[185] So rich meats, poultry, and fish that are full of fat are hotter, moister, more filling, and faster to pass by stool (because moist things pass by stool easier than dry things[186]) than are lean meats, poultry, and fish.[187] Excessive amounts of fat can obstruct the liver and cause indigestion, which is always important to keep in mind.

We can of course modify these thick foods by cooking them in different ways. Boiling makes them more moistening, frying more drying, and baking slightly more drying. So boiled fish offers the thinnest nourishment in a soft, easy to digest form, while fried meat offers the thickest nourishment in a hard, difficult to digest form. Fried meat is most appropriate for

184 Hippocrates 4, Regimen 2, Ch 47-8.
185 Hippocrates 4, Regimen 2, Ch 56. Dioscorides, p219.
186 Hippocrates 4, Regimen 2, Ch 56.
187 Hippocrates 4, Regimen 2, Ch 56.

those who exercise a lot, while boiled fish is most appropriate for those who are sedentary or ill.

Eggs are another nourishing and thick food.[188] They can be prepared in many ways, from being barely cooked at all so that they are still runny, to being fried until they are solid. Barely cooked eggs, which Galen calls 'suckable,' are not very nourishing and pass quickly through the body. At the other end of the spectrum, eggs can be fried, making them extremely hard and thick, being very difficult to digest. From softest to hardest, the forms of cooked eggs are: suckable, soft boiled, hard boiled, baked, and then fried.[189] Soft boiled eggs offer the most balanced nourishment, and poached eggs are a moister version of soft boiled eggs, both being balanced choices.

Eggs can also be separated into egg yolk and egg white. The egg yolk is the fatty part of the egg, which is from where the moistness of eggs comes, while the egg white is the dry part of the egg. So egg whites are a drier form of thick nourishment than whole eggs.

Foods made from milk are also thick nourishment. Milk is a combination of the thin, bitter, laxative whey that is very hot but not very nourishing, and the oily thick part that is hot, constipating, and is thick and very nourishing. Milk is wholesome and nourishing, but the thick portion is thick enough that it can harm the head and the bowels and so shouldn't be overused. Whatever is mixed with the milk brings

---

188 Hippocrates 4, Regimen 2, Ch 50.
189 Food, p173.

out one or the other effect of the milk's properties, making it either more binding or more laxative for the bowels. So mixing milk with coffee, a bitter, thin, purgative food, brings out the laxative effects of the milk, and mixing milk with meat, as for a thick sauce, brings out its binding power.

The thick fat in milk is what makes whole milk moist, while the whey is the component of milk which makes it very heating.[190] Taken together in the form of whole milk, the whey and fat combine to make milk a hot and moist food. Because of the heat, milk, even though it is a liquid, is not good to quench thirst,[191] and because of the high amount of fat, milk can clog the liver and cause indigestion.

When the fat of milk is removed to make lowfat and nonfat milk, it makes the resulting milk hotter by emphasizing the effects of the whey, and it makes it drier by removing the moistening fat. The result is a less nourishing food that is hotter and drier, more appropriate for those who are cold and moist, and for those who are over-nourished/fat.

The opposite is true of foods that concentrate the fatty portion of milk, namely cream and butter. Cream has much less of the whey portion of milk, and thereby becomes a thicker, cooler, moister, and more nourishing food. And butter takes this even further by completely removing the whey from the milk. Butter is thick, very moist, and very nourishing, and it can easily cause obstruction of the liver. It's important to understand that fat is heating and so these foods are by no

---

190 Food, p167.
191 Hippocrates 4, Aphorisms, Ch 5.64.

means cooling, they are just less heating that is whole milk itself.

Milk can also be fermented and made sour, becoming yogurt or cheese. When milk becomes yogurt it neutralizes the hot and bitter power of the whey and takes on a sour flavor, making it cooling. Yogurt has only the fatty part of milk left, and this much colder.[192] So yogurt is cold and moist. This coldness of yogurt can be troublesome to people with cold stomachs, making it difficult to digest,[193] but especially when eaten cold, yogurt can cool a stomach that is too hot.[194]

The fermentation to make cheese from milk is a removal of the moisture in the milk. It is also a process of adding bitterness, which adds heat. So all cheese is drier and hotter than milk. Cheese is a hot, dry, and very nourishing food.[195] It is very thick and slow to pass through the body. The harder the cheese, the more drying it is, the harder is its nourishment, the harder it is to digest, and the thicker is its nourishment. Galen tells us: "You should therefore take special care to avoid [old and harsh] cheese, since it is no good for digestion, assimilation, urination, evacuation of the stomach, or for the healthy state of the [blood]."[196] Fresh cheese is best, avoiding what is old and harsh, because pleasant cheese causes no harm to the stomach and doesn't have any bad juices. Good quality cheese, that is, cheese

---

192 Food, p167.
193 Food, p166.
194 Food, p166.
195 Hippocrates 4, Regimen 2, Ch 51.
196 Food, p169.

that is fresh, soft, and not too harsh to taste, offers reasonably good nourishment that is heating and drying.

Galen gives some good advice about selecting cheeses. He says that all cheese has a consistency that is either soft or hard, dense or porous, glutinous or crumbling, and that it has a taste that is either sharp, bitter, greasy, or sweet. The cheeses with the most balancing nourishment are soft, porous, and midway between glutinous and crumbling, and have no pronounced quality in taste, being a little sweeter than they are sharp, bitter, or greasy. It should also be moderately salty, neither lacking salt nor being extremely salty.

Cottage cheese deserves a special remark. It is at once cheese and yet at the extreme end of softness, moistness, and mildness. It is only slightly hotter, drier, thicker, and more nourishing than whole milk and is a reasonably balancing choice for cheese. When cottage cheese is made from lowfat or nonfat milk, it becomes hotter and drier than cottage cheese made from whole milk.

The following table shows the balance of dairy foods:

	Cold	Moderate	Hot	Hotter
Dry				Cheese
Moderate		Cottage cheese		Lowfat or nonfat milk and cottage cheese
Moist	Yogurt		Whole Milk	
Moister			Butter	

Another type of food that offers thick nourishment is beans. Beans in general offer a good amount of thick nourishment and are soft, passing quickly through the body and causing much flatulence.[197] Peas are not as soft as the other beans, and are therefore the most neutral choice for beans.[198] Garbanzo beans (or chickpeas) are thicker and more nourishing than other beans, making them a more extreme choice of bean,[199] but they pass easily by stool.[200] Lentils are the most extreme of the beans. They are very drying and are appropriate only for those who are too moist.[201] They should not be eaten in the dry time of the year. But mixing them with pearled barley is a good choice, since pearled barley is of the exact opposite nature (cold and moist).

---

197 Food, p98.
198 Food, p99.
199 Food, p100.
200 Hippocrates 4, Regimen 2, Ch 45.
201 Food, p96-8.

Beans are unique among the thick nourishment in that they offer soft, spongy nourishment instead of the hard nourishment that comes from the other thick foods such as meat, poultry, fish, eggs, and cheese. This soft nourishment of beans makes the body softer and spongier as opposed to the hard flesh made by the other thick foods.[202] In this way their effects are more like the thin foods, which in general are soft and make the body softer. In addition, beans pass quickly, which again is unlike the other thick foods. Beans are also flatulent and purgative, but if you grill or bake them they lose this power, become harder to digest, and become a thicker food closer in action to the other thick foods.[203]

Seeds are another form of thick nourishment. Sesame seeds are very thick and hard, and are also very heating. They have strong properties that can be damaging in large quantities. Ideally they are combined with opposite foods in order to decrease their power.[204]

The following chart summarizes the effects of these thick foods:

---

202 Food, p116.
203 Food, p100.
204 Food, p105.

	Cold	Moderate	Hot
Dry			Cheese, fish, sesame seeds, lentils
Moderate		Beans*, seeds*	Poultry
Moist	Yogurt		Meat, milk, eggs

* In general, most beans and seeds are relatively neutral compared to other foods.

Bread and Grains

Grains and bread require a special discussion of their own, for, as Galen succinctly states: "... we use bread all the time."[205] In the ancient world of both the Greeks and Romans, bread was served with every course of every meal. It was the symbol of food itself. So it's important that we understand the power of this important food, starting with the grains from which bread is made.

Grains are made of two basic components: the thick part which is thick, sticky, and extremely nourishing, and the bran which is thin, soft, spongy, and not nourishing at all. The thick portion passes very slowly through the body, while the bran passes through the body very readily.[206] Each grain has a different portion of thick nourishment and bran, making their effects very different.

---

205 Food, p83.
206 Food, p94.

Wheat is the most common of grains. It is hot and dry, and offers a relatively thick nourishment compared to the other grains. Whole wheat has some amount of bran, but its overall thickness is strong enough that it does not pass quickly through the body. It is the gluten in wheat that makes it so thick. Gluten can be helpful or harmful, depending on circumstances. If we need thinner nourishment, then gluten is not helpful at all, but for those who are very active, requiring thick nourishment, and for those who need to thicken their blood, gluten is very helpful.[207] This is yet another example of the wisdom of the ancients. Gluten is neither good nor bad. It is useful for some people at some times and harmful at others.

Rice is mildly hot, dry, and binding to the bowels.[208] It is much like wheat but harder to digest and less nourishing.[209] Rye is hot and dry, like wheat, but easier to digest.[210] Oats strike a balance between their thick nourishment and their bran, making them neither constipating nor laxative.[211] They are therefore less nourishing than wheat because they pass through the body faster. They are cooling and moistening.[212] Millet contains more bran than thick nourishment, and is therefore less nourishing and fairly laxative.[213] It is cold and

---

207 Food, p85.
208 Culpeper, p133.
209 Food, p96.
210 Culpeper, p142.
211 Food, p95.
212 Hippocrates 4, Regimen 2, Ch 43.
213 Food, p95-6.

dry.[214] It is useful to dry a stomach that is too moist.[215] Hippocrates specifically recommends it, mixed with figs, as a strong nourishment for hard workers.[216] Figs (being hot and moist) complement the cool and dry nourishment of the millet, making a nourishing meal that is also cool for those in danger of being overheated through lots of exercise.

Wheat, oats, and millet should be compared in their composition of thick nourishment and bran. Wheat contains the most thick nourishment, and millet the least, with oats striking a balance between these extremes.

But the most important contrast to make is between the two primary grains of the ancient Greeks and Romans: wheat and barley. These two grains are at extreme opposite ends of the spectrum. Wheat is hot, dry, thick, and slow to pass, while barley is cool, moist, much less thick, and quick to pass through the body.[217] Barley suffices for those who take no exercise, but for those who exercise, thicker nourishment is needed.[218] Barley is always cooling, but can be prepared so as to be moistening or drying. Barley that is parched is drying, while pearled barley is moistening when swollen from being boiled.[219]

---

214 Food, p95-6.
215 Food, p96.
216 Hippocrates 4, Regimen 2, Ch 35.
217 Food, p86.
218 Food, p89.
219 Food, p86-7.

The powers of wheat and barley are quite contrasting. Wheat is heating and barley is cooling.[220] So wheat is most appropriate during the cold times of the year, and barley during the hot times. In fact, barley groats can be combined with wine or honeyed wine and drunk during the hot months of the year to quench one's thirst and cool the body.[221]

	Cold	Hot
Dry	Millet	Wheat, rice, rye
Moist	Barley, oats	

Most grains can be made into bread, and there are three main categories of bread: 1) bread made from just the bran which is the least nourishing type of bread and moves very fast through the body; 2) refined bread made from the flour of the grain with the bran removed which is the most nourishing type of bread and moves very slowly through the body; and 3) whole grain bread which is made from both the thick nourishment and the bran which is moderately nourishing and moves at a moderate pace through the body.[222] All breads made from any grain fall into one of these categories.[223]

It's important to understand that ancient people did not have a prejudice against refined foods the way that we modern people do. We've been indoctrinated with the idea that whole grain bread is good and that refined bread is bad. But the ancients did not make such a simplistic, blanket

220 Food, p86.
221 Food, p89.
222 Food, p78-9, 89.
223 Food, p88.

condemnation of refined foods. In fact, refined foods, such as white flour, were considered more nourishing than whole foods because they allowed one to replenish oneself with less bulk. For those who are too lean and undernourished, and for those who live physically-demanding lives, there are few things better than bread made from refined flour for replenishing the body. And refined bread can help to slow digestion. So those whose bowels are too moist, suffering from diarrhea, benefit from refined bread instead of whole grain bread. The following statement from Hippocrates makes it clear just how comfortable these ancient people were with refined foods: "Bread made of [wheat] without separating the bran dries and passes; when cleaned from the bran it nourishes more, but is less laxative."[224] The wisdom demonstrated here should prove extremely useful to our modern lives. Ancient people took great care not to make the world black-and-white, instead maintaining the ability to see the usefulness of many different things.

Galen lists the foods that were commonly used as accompaniments to a dish of bread at the meal. These foods will be discussed in detail in the following section on thin foods. They include: capers, olives, fennel, dill, basil, beets, lettuce, leeks, thyme, savory, oregano, onions, garlic, radish, and mint.[225] These are all foods that make bread more appetizing and digestible and that bread in turn makes more appetizing and digestible.

---

224 Hippocrates 4, Regimen 2, Ch 42.
225 Food, p140, 145, 152.

A discussion of bread is not complete without discussing fatty and sweetened breads such as cakes and donuts. Hippocrates makes their effects quite clear when he says: "All foods from [flour] boiled or fried with honey and oil are heating... very nourishing and do not pass by stool, heating because in one place are fat, sweet and ill-assorted ingredients, which should not be cooked in the same way."[226] Basically, all cakes and fried breads are full of thick juices that are rarely anything but damaging.[227] Breads are often made with a certain amount of butter mixed with the dough. The addition of butter makes the bread hotter, moister, thicker, more filling, and more nourishing than it otherwise would be. These are extreme forms of food that should not routinely be consumed.

We have a number of options for our thick nourishment, mostly from the flesh of animals, but also including eggs, dairy, beans, and grains. Depending on one's activity level, either chicken, pork, or fish, and always bread, are the most balancing choices for thick nourishment.[228] The following table summarizes:

---

226 Hippocrates 4, Regimen 2, Ch 42.
227 Food, p82.
228 Food, p176.

	Cold	Moderate	Hot
Dry	Millet		Cheese, wheat, fish
Moderate		Beans, seeds	Poultry
Moist	Barley, oats		Meat, milk, butter, eggs

Thin Nourishment: Fruits and Vegetables

The nourishment provided by the foods we have so far discussed allow us to easily replenish ourselves, but they come at a price, for their nourishment is thick. Thick foods are hard to digest and can overly thicken our blood. Thin foods give us a chance to balance our meals. By adding thin foods to a meal, the overall thickness of the meal reduces and it therefore becomes easier to digest and more balancing to the blood. Fruits and vegetables make up the large bulk of the thin foods. They also have wonderful powers to heat, cool, dry, and moisten the body, making these thin foods our best way of helping to keep our meals balancing for our health. As we discuss these thin foods we should bear in mind that they should almost always be served before thick foods or combined with them. Galen says to "eat all vegetables [thin foods] before other foods."[229]

In general, fruit relaxes the body and softens the flesh.[230] Fruit is thin, soft, and digests quickly and easily. Although fruit

229 Hygiene, p216.
230 Hippocrates 4, Regimen 2, Ch 40-56.

digests quickly, it does not easily assimilate into the flesh of the body, creating a significant amount of waste material. However, ripe fruit is much less harmful than unripe fruit,[231] unripe fruit being useful only for replenishing moisture after prolonged labor,[232] and overripe fruit being only useful as a food which passes extremely quickly through the body.

Although all fruit has a degree of unwholesomeness, figs have less unwholesomeness than all other fruits, pass quickly through the body, and purge the bowels.[233] Their nourishment is thin, but they are more nourishing than other fruit. Like all fruit, they make soft, spongy flesh. In this way they are similar to beans. Galen is careful to point out that perfectly ripe figs and dried figs cause almost no harm, although eating too many can cause harm. Fresh figs are hot and moist, and dried figs are hotter and less moist. Dried figs are a great appetizer. When mixed with a fatty food, such as walnuts, they help the liver to handle thicker foods.[234] Galen summarizes the power of figs and grapes by saying, "Figs and grapes are what one might call the chief of the autumn fruits. They nourish more than all the other autumn fruits and they contain fewer bad juices, especially when they are fully ripe."[235]

---

231 Food, p116.
232 Food, p111.
233 Food, p115-6.
234 Food, p116.
235 Food, p117.

Grapes nourish less than figs but pass more quickly through the body.[236] The power of grapes differs by their flavor, those that are sweet are heating and cause thirst, while those that are sour are cold, and those that are more neutral in their flavor are neither heating nor cooling. Fresh grapes are moist,[237] and raisins are hotter and less moist.[238] As can be gleaned from what has already been said, dried fruit is a hotter, drier, more nourishing, and thicker form of the fresh fruit.[239]

Dates are similar to both figs and grapes. Much like raisins, their power can be ascertained by their flavor, the sweeter dates being hot and the sour dates being cold.

Plums are another relatively wholesome fruit that, when ripe, does little harm to the body.[240] They are cold and moist, and their cooling power makes them a good alternative to figs when cooling instead of heating is desired. In dried form they are warmer and drier as prunes.

Citrus fruits all carry a strong sour flavor. The juice of lemons and limes has a very strong sour flavor and so should be treated as a seasoning instead of as a food. Their juice is cool and dry, offers no nourishment, and slows digestion. It stimulates the appetite, and so lemon or lime juice is excellent when used to season appetizers. The sour flavor strengthens

---

236 Food, p117.
237 Hippocrates 4, Regimen 2, Ch 55.
238 Hippocrates 4, Regimen 2, Ch 55.
239 Hippocrates 4, Regimen 2, Ch 56.
240 Food, p133.

the stomach and helps it to digest foods better, and so foods seasoned with lemon or lime juice are easier to digest. The danger of lemon and lime juice is that if it is used too heavily it can thicken food to such a degree that it causes indigestion and upsets the stomach. So lemon and lime juice is a great seasoning, but like all seasonings can be overused and cause problems.

Oranges are similar to lemons and limes, but oranges have less sour and more sweet flavor, making them more nourishing, less cooling, and less drying. Oranges are a mildly sour food offering a thin nourishment.

Melons are cooling, moistening, diuretic, and pass quickly.[241] Cantaloupe and honeydew pose no serious problems for digestion, but watermelons are extreme forms of melons.[242] They are more cooling and moistening and pass extremely quickly through the body. They can cause significant digestive irritation if eaten alone. They should be combined with foods that have good juices, such as lettuce. Melons make excellent appetizers.

All gourds such as pumpkin, butternut squash, and acorn squash are warm, moistening, thin, and pass quickly through the body.[243] They warm because of their sweet flavor, but in general these foods are fairly neutral and take on the power of whatever is used to season them.[244]

---

241 Food, p114.
242 Food, p113.
243 Hippocrates 4, Regimen 2, Ch 54.
244 Food, p112.

Cucumbers are cold and moist.[245]

Apricots, peaches, and nectarines are extremely thin nourishment and pass through the body very quickly.[246] They rot and cause indigestion if they are not made to pass very rapidly[247] and so should be eaten before other foods. They are hot and moist.

Apples can be primarily sweet, bitter, or sour, but no matter what they all carry a strong sour flavor, so they are all cooling and drying, and they all slow the digestion of a meal.[248] Sour apples are the most cooling and drying, sweet apples the least, and bitter apples are warmer than sour apples.

Apples serve as a great final course to meals, thickening the end of the meal with their sour flavor. Through their sour flavor, apples strengthen the stomach and help it to function better.[249] Bitter apples also carry the power of the bitter flavor to cut through thick juices. They can be used to move the bowels when thick foods have clogged the bowels.

Baked apples are easier to digest than raw apples. Baked apples served with bread after a meal will strengthen the stomach and bowels for those who have lost their appetite, for those who are slow to digest their food, and for those suffering from vomiting or diarrhea. Hippocrates says: "Apple

---

245 Food, p115.
246 Food, p124.
247 Food, p115-6.
248 Food, p126.
249 Food, p125-8.

juice stops vomiting... [and the] smell too of apples is good for vomiting."[250]

Pears are almost the same as apples, but warmer, moister, and more nourishing.[251] They are similarly powered as apples, and pear juice works much like apple juice. So the major difference is that pears are warmer and moister and are thus more appropriate for those who are cold and dry, and pears are more nourishing than apples and so are more appropriate for those who need more nourishment.

Olives are bitter and therefore heating and move quickly through the bowels. They are thin nourishment and make a great appetizer by strengthening the stomach and whetting the appetite.[252] Olives that are preserved in vinegar are cooler and dryer, and those preserved in salt are hotter and dryer.

Pickled capers are neutral and devoid of nourishment. They relax the bowels, whet the appetite, cleanse the stomach, bring up phlegm, and purge blockages of the liver and spleen. For all these reasons they make excellent appetizers.[253]

Olive oil has a bitter flavor and thus has a purgative and drying power that balances the fatty, moistening, nourishing power that it also possesses. It mixes well with many foods to help them to pass through the body more readily. Olive oil must be compared and contrasted to butter. Butter is the moist portion of milk. It is fat and sweet and therefore very

250 Hippocrates 4, Regimen 2, Ch 55.
251 Hippocrates 4, Regimen 2, Chapter 55. Food, p129-30.
252 Food, p131.
253 Food, p134.

heating, but it has no bitter flavor like olive oil, so it doesn't speed its way through the bowels. Butter is moist while olive oil has a drying power, and butter is extremely nourishing while olive oil is only nourishing if it passes slowly. Butter, being more nourishing and moistening, is more appropriate for those who are undernourished and/or dry, while olive oil, which includes a cleansing and purgative element, is more appropriate for those who are over-nourished and/or moist.

Berries are thin nourishment appropriate as appetizers. The sweet ones are heating and the sour ones cooling. They all moisten to a certain extent. Mulberries warm and moisten.[254] Mulberries pass extremely quickly and so should be eaten first so that they don't rot. They prepare the body for other foods.[255] They are great when the stomach and or liver is too hot and dry.

Strawberries are cool and moist.[256]

Lettuce is praised by Galen as being one of the few foods to have almost no negative impact on the body. It is converted almost directly into blood.[257] It is mildly cooling and moistening.[258] It can cool a stomach that is too hot, and it helps with insomnia if eaten in the evening.[259] Lettuce is best

---

254 Hippocrates 4, Regimen 2, Ch 55.
255 Food, p122.
256 Culpeper, p173.
257 Food, p139.
258 Hippocrates 4, Regimen 2, Ch 40-56.
259 Food, p139.

served with something mildly bitter such as celery, leek, or basil, which helps to balance it completely.

Spinach is cool and moist.[260]

Beets are bitter and so heating. They offer almost no nourishment at all and are a very thin food. They help to purge the stomach and bowels, and especially when taken with mustard or vinegar they help obstructions of the liver and spleen.

Cabbage is a powerful food. It warms and dries the body.[261] Ancient doctors used it as a drying medicine, and so it should be cooked so as not to cause excessive drying. Cooked cabbage helps to move the bowels.[262] Culpeper has this to say about cabbage: "They are most commended being eaten before meat to keep one from surfeiting [overeating], as also from being drunk with too much wine, and quickly makes a drunken man sober; for as they say, there is such an antipathy and enmity between the vine and the colewort [cabbage], that the one will die where the other groweth."[263]

Galen and Hippocrates both discuss how cabbage can be used as a medicine.[264] It is the juice of the cabbage that helps to move the bowels, and the flesh of the cabbage that is drying.[265] To separate the juice and the flesh, one boils the

---

260 Culpeper, p161.
261 Food, p140-1.
262 Hippocrates 4, Regimen 2, Ch 54.
263 Culpeper, p31.
264 Hippocrates 4, Regimen 2, Ch 54.
265 Food, p140-1.

cabbage. The flesh is then removed from the water in which its juice has now been mixed. The remaining flesh can be boiled once again in fresh water in order to make a very drying medicine, while the original boiled water, which contains much of the juice of the cabbage, can be drunk as a very cleansing medicine that helps to remove excessively hot and dry matter from the body. Taken as a food, raw cabbage is hot and very drying, and cooked cabbage less drying.

Garlic and onions are both extremely powerful foods. They are very bitter, heating, and drying, and they pass through the body very rapidly.[266] These foods are more like purging medicines than foods, but they are wonderful seasonings and should be treated as such.[267] They offer essentially no nourishment to the body.[268] They thin any foods with which they come in contact, and so can help to make any thick food less troublesome to digest. Garlic in particular is a very powerful remedy for constipation[269] because of its purging power. But care should be taken here, because bowels that are too hot and too dry are often constipated, and garlic can make such bowels even hotter and drier. So garlic should only be used to help with constipated bowels that are not too hot and dry.

When any food is cooked, especially for a long period of time, it loses its power. And this is a very useful thing to know about garlic and onions, for their power is so great that they

---

266 Hippocrates 4, Regimen 2, Ch 40-56.
267 Food, p152.
268 Hippocrates 4, Regimen 2, Ch 40-56.
269 Food, p152.

can easily cause imbalances. They should almost never be eaten raw, but instead should be at least mildly cooked, and often cooked a great deal.[270]

Radishes are bitter, hot, and moist.[271] They have the power to cut through and eliminate excessively cold matter in the body.[272] Radishes eaten raw can be excessively heating and cause indigestion, so they are best eaten seasoned with vinegar or accompanied by bread.[273] Radishes move through the body very quickly and thus serve well as appetizers. Thin slices of radish on bread is a nice appetizer for cold and dry people.

Celery is a relatively neutral food. It is slightly bitter and therefore slightly heating.[274] Galen recommends that we mix it with lettuce to balance the slight cooling power of lettuce in order to form a very well-balanced dish.[275] Celery is also pleasant for the stomach and is one of the few foods that does essentially no harm.[276]

Carrots and turnips are harder to digest than other thin foods.[277] A course of either one should be eaten near the end of the thin part of the meal, since the power of these foods are more like thick nourishment than the other thin foods.

---

270 Food, p124.
271 Food, p152.
272 Hippocrates 4, Regimen 2, Ch 40-56.
273 Food, p152.
274 Food, p144.
275 Food, p144.
276 Food, p143.
277 Food, p148, p151.

Carrots and turnips are both heating and moistening,[278] the carrot hotter and thinner than the turnip.

Asparagus is cold and dry.[279] It has a sour flavor that is good for the stomach.[280] Artichokes similarly benefit the stomach and should be boiled and served with olive oil.[281]

Mushrooms, especially when boiled, come close to a flavorless food. Their nourishment is cold and moist, and can cause us to become too cold and moist if overeaten.[282]

Nuts in general are more nourishing than other thin foods due to the fat that they contain, and this fat makes them heating.[283] Pine nuts are one of the thickest of the thin foods. They are nutritious, hard to digest, and are a well-balanced nourishment for the body.[284] Walnuts and hazelnuts are very useful. They have enough fat to relax the bowels and enough sour flavor to strengthen the stomach,[285] which combines to make them relatively neutral in their power to heat, cool, dry, or moisten the body. Almonds are unique in that they have almost no degree of sour flavor. Their bitter flavor gives them the power to thin any thick juices in the body.[286] They are hot

---

278 Hippocrates 4, Regimen 2, Ch 54.
279 Hippocrates 4, Regimen 2, Ch 40-56.
280 Food, p146.
281 Food, p143.
282 Food, p151.
283 Hippocrates 4, Regimen 2, Ch 55.
284 Food, p124.
285 Food, p132.
286 Food, p132.

and nourishing,[287] but not as nourishing as walnuts.[288] Pistachios are not very nourishing, but they strengthen the liver by purging the juices that block its passages, having a quality that is bitter and sour.[289] Nuts can be ground into nut butters, which makes them viscous and slow to pass through the body. Nut butters can easily cause blockages of the liver. They are extremely nourishing. The following table illustrates the power of thin foods.

---

287 Hippocrates 4, Regimen 2, Ch 55.
288 Food, p132.
289 Food, p133.

	Cold	Moderate	Hot
Dry	Asparagus, artichoke, pickles, lemons, limes, oranges, apples, pears		Onion, garlic, cabbage, beet, olive oil
Moderate	Prunes	Lettuce, celery, capers, pine nuts, walnuts, hazelnuts, pistachios winter squash	Olives, almonds
Moist	Sour grapes, plums, strawberries, sour berries, melons, cucumbers, spinach, mushrooms		Radish, carrot, turnip, figs, sweet grapes, raisins, sweet berries, apricots, peaches, nectarines

Seasonings and Sweeteners

The sweet flavor is heating and so all sweeteners are heating. Honey was the main sweetener in the ancient world of

Hippocrates. When raw, it warms and dries due to its underlying bitter flavor,[290] which also makes it move through the body quickly and thus nourishes very little.[291] When cooked, however, honey loses its bitter flavor and thus moves slowly through the body and nourishes much.[292] Honey has such a heating power that it easily imbalances those who are too hot, but it is extremely useful for those who are too cold.[293] When raw honey is mixed with water its power is tempered, making this a useful drink to help to moisten those whose bowels are too hot and too dry, relieving constipation, and also to stop diarrhea by warming and drying the bowels of those whose bowels are too cold and too moist.[294] Honeyed water is thus a useful drink for almost everyone.

Other sweeteners are quite different than honey, most lacking the bitter flavor of honey and thus lacking any power to dry or evacuate the bowels. They are very nourishing, and they are all heating and can cause inflammation of the liver.

The sugar from sugarcane helps the stomach and bowels.[295] It has three forms: white sugar, brown sugar, and molasses. White sugar is highly-refined and devoid of everything but the sweet flavor. Because white sugar is so highly-refined, it has lost all trace of the original food from which it is derived, and thus offers us nothing but heat. It can easily inflame the liver

---

290 Food, p186-8.
291 Food, p67.
292 Food, p186-8.
293 Food, p186-8.
294 Hippocrates 4, Regimen 2, Ch 40-56.
295 Dioscorides, p226.

and spleen, and it does nothing to move the bowels. There is a big difference between refined sugar and refined flour, for the power of the wheat is not removed from the refined flour. We need to recognize the difference between the ancient form of refinement, which is simply the removal of part of a food, and the modern form of refinement of sugar. Refined flour has its healthful uses, while refined sugar is simply dangerous and extreme, completely removing the original food itself. Molasses is the thick, sticky substance that collects at the bottom when white sugar is being cooked out of the sugarcane. It is where all the parts of the sugarcane plant itself collects, and is thus a concentrated form of the plant. It is viscous and slower to pass through the body, and it has the greatest power to help the stomach and bowels. Brown sugar is a mixed form of white sugar and molasses, carrying a mixture of their powers.

Herbs and spices have powerful medicinal powers which will be discussed in detail in the chapter *Herbs and Remedies for Balance*. In general, almost all herbs and spices are drying. Onions, garlic, leeks, fennel, dill, coriander/cilantro, pepper, ginger, thyme, sage, marjoram/oregano, savory, and basil are all drying.[296] When used to season foods these seasonings make the dish remarkably more drying.

Basil is specifically warned against by the ancients as having bad juices that can injure the stomach and is itself hard to digest.[297] So we should be careful about basil.

---

296 Food, p144-5, 158. Hippocrates 4, Regimen 2, Ch 54.
297 Food, p145.

Pepper and ginger are specifically mentioned for their ability to cut and dissolve foods, making food easier to digest.[298] We should make good use of them in our meals to assist our digestion.

Vinegar

Vinegar is sour and thus cooling and drying. Hippocrates calls it refreshing because it dissolves and consumes the moisture in the body.[299] It is less drying than wine.[300] Vinegar is basically wine, which is hot and dry, that has taken on a sour flavor, which makes it cold and dry. Vinegar doesn't nourish the body at all, which makes it a seasoning or a medicine, not really a food.[301]

Pickles

Pickling involves preserving foods in both salt and vinegar. Galen says that "... the power of salt... is such as to dissipate, through attenuation and absorption, excessive moisture in those bodies with which it has contact."[302] Essentially, salt dries the food preserved in it. Vinegar, with its sour flavor, also has a drying power. Salt is heating and the sour flavor of vinegar is cooling, which essentially cancel each other out on the hot and cold spectrum. But both salt and sour are drying, which makes pickles a much drier version of the original food. For example, cucumbers, which are a cool and moist food,

---

298 Hygiene, p158.
299 Hippocrates 4, Regimen 2, Ch 40-56.
300 Hippocrates 4, Regimen 2, Ch 56.
301 Food, p67.
302 Food, p189.

become cool and dry when pickled. Pickled versions of foods are also easier to digest than their original form.[303] So pickles are drier and easier to digest than their former version.

Drinks

Foods replenish the solid parts of the body that melt away during the day, and drinks replenish the liquid that is lost. Water is cold and moist,[304] and alcohol is hot and dry.[305] Water is most appropriate during the hot and dry times of the year, and alcohol is more appropriate during the cold and moist times of the year.

The hot and dry power of alcohol is extremely heating and can fill the head with hot fumes. Those who are too hot must be extremely careful with alcohol because it can easily imbalance them toward heat. But alcohol also has the power to soften and thin excessively thick juices in the body. It promotes the elimination of waste through perspiration and urine.[306] In particular, thin white wines promote urine the most.[307] The thicker the wine, the thicker is its nourishment. Red, thick wine, is the hardest to digest and the most nourishing, and thin, white wine is the thinnest and least nourishing. Sweet wines are hotter and easier to digest than dry wines,[308] but are also even hotter than other wines because of the heat generated by the sweet flavor.

303 Hippocrates 4, Regimen 2, Ch 56. Food, p186.
304 Hippocrates 4, Regimen 2, Ch 40-56.
305 Hippocrates 4, Regimen 2, Ch 40-56.
306 Hygiene, p34.
307 Hygiene, p204.
308 Food, p188-9.

Juice that is sweet is heating and moistening, and juice that is sour is cooling and drying. Sweetening a sour juice, as with lemonade, neutralizes the sour flavor so that it is relatively neutral in its power. Bitter drinks, such as tea and coffee, are heating and drying. When sweetened these drinks becomes even more heating. The following chart makes the effects of various common drinks clear.

	Cold	Moderate	Hot
Dry		Mild tea with lemon	Alcohol, bitter tea/coffee
Moderate	Water with lemon	Mild tea	Sweetened tea/coffee
Moist	Water		Milk

Sweetening a drink moves it toward the Hot/Moist side of the chart. Adding a sour flavor, such as adding lemon juice, moves it toward the Cold/Dry side. Making it bitter (such as steeping tea in water) moves it toward the Hot/Dry side. And diluting it with water moves it toward the Cold/Moist side. These are very useful rules for understanding the effects of our drinks.

Seasonal and Constitutional Eating

All of these details about food can seem overwhelming, so it is good to remember this simple advice from Galen: "... soft and [easily broken down[309]] food is best for the maintenance

---

309 Grant's introduction to Food.

of health, because it is the most wholesome of all. For guaranteed health, there is no better way than through wholesomeness."[310] That is, foods that are easily digested and most easily assimilated into the flesh and blood of our bodies, such as chicken, fish, bread, lettuce, figs, and grapes are the foods that should most routinely be found at our tables.[311] If we emphasize these foods, then it's hard to go wrong.

Besides the wholesomeness of our meals, we want to be mindful of using foods that will help to keep us balanced. Those with a hot constitution should almost always emphasize slightly cooling foods, while those who have a cold constitution should do the opposite. Likewise, those with a moist constitution should emphasize dry foods, and those who are dry should emphasize moist foods. The same is true during the cycle of the seasons, with hotter foods more appropriate during the cold times of the year and cold foods more appropriate during the warm months. Galen tells us:

> With each foodstuff you must be aware of locality, season and climate, in autumn being abstemious with foods that are drying, but using them in winter, just as of course in summer using foods that are moist and cooling. But in spring, which is average in its temperament, foods that are average in their powers should be served. Yet there is no single category of average foods. For some of these foods generally have something in common with the extremes, whilst some a

---

310 Food, p181.
311 Food, p176.

central position through two things of equal power being blended....[312]

Bearing this in mind, let's discuss how a meal can be altered in order to make it more balancing for various people under various circumstances.

First, we should remember that those who are excessively moist can become more dry by taking fewer meals (one meal per day), and those who are too dry can become more moist by taking more meals (two or even three meals per day).

There are a number of foods to choose from as appetizers. Some of them are heating and others are cooling, some of them are moistening and others drying, and some of them are relatively neutral in their effect. The following table helps to illustrate the effects of common appetizers:

	Cold	Moderate	Hot
Dry	Pickled cucumbers		Olive in salt
Moderate	Cucumbers	Capers	Olives in vinegar, dried figs
Moist	Melons		Radish, fresh figs

It makes sense to start a meal with olives preserved in salt during the cold and moist times of the year, and to start a meal with melon during the hot and dry times of the year. And

312 Food, p98.

a person with a hot and moist constitution should rarely if ever start a meal with radishes, for example, while a cold and dry person should avoid pickles.

After the appetizer, one should begin drinking. Water or mild tea is appropriate for almost everyone at this part of the meal.

After the appetizer comes the thin nourishment. This can consist of a number of courses of vegetables and/or fruits, and those vegetables and/or fruits can be prepared in many ways so as to modify their effects on the balance of the body, so there are many options for the thin nourishment of a meal. The following table and a few examples should help to illustrate:

	Cold	Moderate	Hot
Dry	Baked asparagus	Celery	Sauteed Cabbage
Moderate	Oranges	Lettuce and celery	Baked carrots
Moist	Raw plums	Lettuce	Boiled carrots

Someone who is currently well-balanced might choose to have lettuce and celery, which combine together in a very balanced way. Someone who is too cold and too moist might choose sauteed cabbage. Someone who is too hot and too dry might choose to eat raw plums.

Another round of drinking should occur during and after the thin nourishment. Those who are too hot or too dry should probably stick with water, while those who are too cold or too moist may want to begin having some alcohol at this time in order to help to heat and to dry. It's important to understand that the ancients drank alcohol frequently, and so both Hippocrates and Galen make it seem rare to do otherwise. This is not to encourage those who don't drink to suddenly start drinking, but only to remain faithful to what Hippocrates says. A bitter tea is another option to help to heat and dry.

After the thin nourishment, it is time for the main course of thick nourishment. This can consist of a number of courses of meat, poultry, fish, eggs, dairy, beans, and/or grains, although often will consist of just one main dish. This main course should of course be prepared in such a way as to modify it to be as balancing as possible. The following chart and examples should help to make this clear:

	Cold	Moderate	Hot
Dry	Millet	Roasted chicken	Baked fish
Moderate		Baked chicken	Baked meat
Moist	Barley	Boiled chicken	Boiled meat

Someone who is currently well-balanced might choose to have baked chicken. Someone who is too cold and too moist might choose baked fish. Someone who is too hot and too dry might choose to eat barley.

Another round of drinking should occur during and after the thick nourishment. Those who are too hot or too dry may want to stick with water, while those who are too cold or too moist should probably have some alcohol or tea at this time in order to help to heat and to dry.

After the thick nourishment it is very helpful to eat something sour in order to thicken the final foods of the meal and help to stimulate the process of digestion. Apples are a very dynamic and useful choice for this part of the meal. The following table should help to illustrate how apples can be used to close a meal.

	Cold	Moderate	Hot
Dry	Baked sour apples		Baked bitter apples
Moderate		Boiled sour apple	
Moist	Raw sweet apples		Boiled sweet apples

Someone who is currently well-balanced might choose to have boiled sour apples. Someone who is too cold and too moist might choose baked bitter apples. Someone who is too hot and too dry might choose to eat raw sweet apples.

All that remains is to discuss the final foods eaten purely for pleasure. As long as these are eaten slowly and in small quantities, and as long as they are not extremely powerful foods, they are not likely to imbalance a person very much. The drinking continues at this time, with the food portion more of an accompaniment to the drinking. Except for those who are extremely imbalanced toward heat or dryness, most people should have some alcohol or a stronger drink at this time, though it's important to note that Hippocrates, Galen, and Culpeper all specifically speak against drunkenness and drinking to excess.

So a reasonably well-balanced person might have the following meal:

- Appetizer: whole wheat bread with capers followed by water;
- Thin Course: lettuce mixed with celery followed by white wine;
- Thick Course: baked chicken followed by red wine;
- Sour Course: boiled sour apples;
- Side Dish: small bites of cheese with red wine.

During the cold and moist time of the year, this same person might change this meal to the following:

- Appetizer: whole wheat bread with salt-preserved olives followed by white wine;
- Thin Course: baked carrots seasoned with garlic followed by white wine;
- Thick Course: baked fish followed by red wine;

- Sour Course: baked bitter apples;
- Side Dish: small bites of cheese with red wine.

During the hot and dry time of the year, this same person might change this meal to the following:

- Appetizer: barley bread with honeydew followed by water;
- Thin Course: lettuce followed by water;
- Thick Course: boiled chicken followed by water;
- Sour Course: raw sweet apples;
- Side Dish: small bites of cheese with white wine.

The following table shows examples of how a person with each constitution might modify the basic meal above for their own needs:

	Hot and Moist	Hot and Dry	Cold and Dry	Cold and Moist
Appetizer	Pickled cucumbers	Melons	Radishes	Olives in salt
Thin Course	Baked asparagus	Raw plums	Boiled carrots	Baked carrots
Thick Course	Millet	Barley	Boiled meat	Baked fish
Sour Course	Baked sour apples	Raw sweet apples	Boiled sweet apples	Baked bitter apples

These are examples only, meant to guide beginners in how to eat as Hippocrates would say. One should read through the food section many times to get a sense of how other foods can be used.

Digestive Problems

There are a number of common digestive problems that can be caused by one of two things, either an imbalanced organ of digestion (the stomach or bowels), or by poor eating habits. When suffering from digestive problems, the first thing that we should consider is our eating habits, how we prepare our foods and how we order them in our meals, and only then consider an imbalance of our stomach or bowels. We will deal with imbalances of the organs in the chapter *Herbs and Remedies for Balance*. For now, we will focus on how we can change our eating habits.

Symptoms of poor digestion include a heavy feeling in the belly, belching, bloating, flatulence, diarrhea, and constipation. All of these can be caused by a liver that is obstructed, which prevents it from helping in the digestion of food, in particular thick foods. The liver becomes obstructed by excess amounts of fat and sweet foods in the diet. Appetizers are extremely helpful for the liver, and so should be our first choice in managing an obstructed liver.[313] Eating dried fruit mixed with a bitter herb such as thyme, pepper, ginger, pennyroyal, savory, calamint, oregano, or hyssop (each having a purgative power), as an appetizer helps to open the liver.[314] A good example is dried figs. The effect of dried fruit is even better when mixed with a fatty food such as

313 Hygiene, p254. Food, p83.
314 Food, p116.

nuts. Galen recommends dried figs mixed with walnuts or almonds for this purpose. Beets are another food with the power to open the liver, especially when seasoned with mustard and vinegar. Pistachios are another option, strengthening the liver and opening its passages.[315]

Many foods create flatulence even if properly prepared and eaten in combination with a well-balanced meal, but this effect can be reduced through cooking. Galen says that "... with all foods any tendency towards flatulence is mitigated through heating and diluting."[316] By thoroughly cooking foods, diluting them in liquids and mixing them with other foods, and by mixing them with bitter foods such as onions, we can reduce their flatulent properties and make digestion easier.

Constipation can be caused by excessively dry bowels, but it can also be caused from eating a meal that is excessively thick and hard to digest. Eating thinner foods and moist foods will help. Following a meal with a gentle walk is very helpful, "...[meals] slide [down the digestive tract] more easily when shaken than if one reclines without moving."[317] Galen says: "It is obvious that drinking sweet wine after eating plums contributes to the evacuation of the bowels, provided that an elapse of time is allowed and [food] is not taken immediately after them. This should be remembered as a basic rule with everything that relaxes the bowels...."[318] The ancient cure for

---

315 Food, p133.
316 Food, p99-100.
317 Food, p72-3.
318 Food, p133.

constipation was thin foods, especially fruit, followed by sweet wine and a gentle walk.

Diarrhea or loose stools can be caused by just the opposite: eating a meal that is excessively thin and easy to digest, having too many vegetables, fruits, oil, or bitter foods. So when suffering with loose stools, one should have thicker foods, less vegetables and fruits, less oil and bitter foods, and should rest after a meal.

For those with any digestive problems, Galen recommends mixing food with a blend of milk and honey, which will help to digest any food with which it is mixed.[319]

Excessive thirst can be caused by an imbalance of the stomach or lungs and will be discussed more thoroughly in the chapter *Herbs and Remedies for Balance*. But when this happens, Hippocrates recommends diminishing both food and fatigue, and drinking diluted wine as cold as possible.[320]

Final Thoughts on Eating

Before we end our discussion of food we must talk about the importance of the quality of our foods and of the art of cooking, for these were of no small importance to the ancients. Hippocrates tells us that fresh foods give more strength,[321] and Galen tells us that unripe foods are more productive of waste and are less nourishing.[322]

---

319 Food, p73.
320 Hippocrates 4, Regimen of Health, Ch 7.
321 Hippocrates 4, Regimen 2, Ch 56.
322 Food, p99.

Ancient people recognized the importance of the quality of their food: "Every animal that feeds off grass sprouting from the ground or the branches and shoots of trees, in the season when their growth is luxuriant, grows more healthy, fattens up and is very suitable to eat."[323] It seems that the 'grass-fed' and 'cage-free' movements of today would have been strongly supported by the ancients. In fact, both Hippocrates and Galen discussed these topics at length, Hippocrates[324] having similar things to say as Galen does in the following passage:

> For the flesh of mullets [a type of fish] which live in water that is muddy and dirty is excrementitious and rather slimy, whilst the flesh of mullets that live in the clear sea is excellent, particularly when the sea is whipped up by the wind. On the subject of calm and waveless sea, the less fish are exercised, the worse their flesh, so they are inferior when they live in what are called lagoons, and still worse when they are in lakes....
>
> Fish become better and worse according to their diet. Some thrive on weeds and lots of excellent roots which makes them superior, whilst others eat slimy weeds and unwholesome roots. Others again which live in rivers that flow through a big city, feeding off human sewage and similarly unpleasant food, are the worst of all, as I have said, so that, if they are left out dead for a short time, they immediately putrefy and smell disgusting. ...
>
> Since these are the worst, the best are the complete opposite, their habitat - as I was saying - being the cleanest sea....

---

323 Food, p155.
324 Hippocrates 4, Regimen 2, Ch 56.

As I have said, it is important to bear in mind with all fish the following common denominator: that the worst fish are nurtured at the mouths of every river that flushes toilets, kitchens, baths, the dirt of clothes and linen, and everything else that is to do with the city that they run through which must be washed away, and especially when the city is densely populated.[325]

It is clear that the ancients cared deeply for the quality of their foods.

Equally important to the ancients were the culinary arts: "Indeed, I do not consider it right for a doctor to be completely ignorant of the art of cooking, because whatever tastes good is easier to digest than other dishes which may be equally as healthy."[326] Bland, oily food was simply not acceptable: "The taste also serves as an immediate indication [of more wholesome food] because the flesh is more full of flavor, pleasant and without any oiliness. Oily foods that are bland in taste are not only worse to eat, but are also more difficult to digest as they are bad for the stomach and unwholesome."[327] We need to select and prepare our foods so that they are appetizing, not oily: "Things that are oily and sticky from the outset fill us up quickly and ruin the appetite, while we cannot bear eating them for many days in a row."[328]

Hippocrates speaks of the importance of the art of cooking: "Raw things cause colic and belching, because what ought to

---

325 Food, p174-179.
326 Food, p131.
327 Food, p175.
328 Food, p177.

be digested by the fire is dealt with by the belly, which is too weak for the substances that enter it."[329] And Galen complains about the digestive problems created by poor cooking: "The common habit of chefs to use unsuitable seasonings in large quantities is such as to cause dyspepsia more than good digestion."[330]

The art of cooking is important for health, because better tasting food is better for the body. And we must bear in mind that the greatest cuisines in the West, those of the French and Italian, are the direct descendants of the culinary arts of the Romans, from where Galen is speaking to us, which in turn is the direct descendant of the culinary arts developed in ancient Greece: the world of Hippocrates. Jeff Smith, known as the Frugal Gourmet, writes: "Greece has been in the forefront of creative cooking since Athena called forth the olive tree in Athens."[331] These ancient people knew a thing or two about taste.

Homer, Plato, Aristotle, Aesop, and Aristophanes all spoke much about food as they discussed art, history, and philosophy. The word 'gastronomy' is the ancient Greek word meaning the practice and study of good eating. By the time of Alexander the Great (the fourth century BC), the Greek culinary art was highly sophisticated, with one of the earliest recorded cookbooks being written by Archestratus at that

---

329 Hippocrates 4, Regimen 2, Ch 56.
330 Food, p144.
331 Smith. *The Frugal Gourmet Cooks Three Ancient Cuisines*. New York: William Morrow and Company, Inc, 1989. P66.

time. It was the desire for a continuous supply of olive oil that led to the development of the Greek navy in order to keep shipping lanes open, which in turn led to the power of the Greek empire, spreading their culture throughout the Mediterranean. One could argue that if the Greeks weren't so focused on the art of cooking, our entire world would be drastically different, and the ancient Greek culture would be long forgotten, instead of the foundation of our entire civilization. The culinary arts were so important in ancient Greece that chefs were given exclusive rights to any recipe they invented for a full year, allowing them to grow very wealthy if they created something so tasty that everyone just had to try it.

When the Greek empire fell and the Romans took control of the Mediterranean, it became extremely popular to live like the ancient Greeks. Galen's deep reverence for Hippocrates is a result of the popularity of ancient Greek civilization in the Roman world. To eat like the ancient Greeks was the fantasy at work in much of the development of the Roman culinary art. Greek cooks were brought into Roman households to run the kitchens.

Lorenza de'Medici, writing about the wonders of Italian cooking, says: "Credit must be given to the ancient Romans for developing the [Italian] peninsula's first culinary tradition, based on the Greek and Etruscan foundations of their civilization."[332] The conquering Romans brought the grape

---

332 de'Medici. *The Heritage of Italian Cooking*. London: Limited Editions, 1993. P11.

vine for wine and the olive tree for oil to what would eventually be France, establishing the foundation of French cooking.[333] Jeff Smith summarizes the culinary heritage of the ancient Greeks and Romans:

> [The ancient Greeks] taught us to make mayonnaise, baked pasta, basic white sauce (Bechamel), fancy breads, the frying pan as we know it today, the stewing pot brought to perfection, the Dutch oven, and the packed lunch. They even taught us to dip our bread in wine, though the Italians and French think it is their custom. Finally, the Romans took a whole style of cuisine from the Greeks, made some wonderful improvements upon it, and then, through their wild and warring travels, took this cuisine to the rest of Europe. When Catherine de Medicis moved to Paris in 1533 to marry Henri II she brought her Florentine cooks with her. The cooking of Paris was radically changed.... The French really did not learn to cook until the beginning of the seventeenth century, and they are not embarrassed by that fact. They admit that the Greeks taught the Romans to cook and the Romans taught the French.[334]

The great cuisines of today are the direct descendants of the cuisine of the ancient Greeks. Galen was not only a doctor but also a man who took the art of cooking very seriously. He was known to have a large collection of recipe books in his possession which he consulted on a regular basis. What would Hippocrates say? He says to learn how to cook! The epigraph for this chapter makes it clear. It is worth repeating here: "[The power of food] is probably the most important of

333 de'Medici. *The Heritage of French Cooking*. New York: Random House, 1991. P11.

334 Smith. *The Frugal Gourmet Cooks Three Ancient Cuisines*. New York: William Morrow and Company, Inc, 1989. P11.

all medical subjects."[335] Food is of paramount importance and proper cooking is the key to its healthy and delightful use.

---

335 Food, p68.

Sleeping for Balance

When he has bathed and eaten, let him sleep
Softly: this is the privilege of age.[336] - Anonymous

Sleep is the primary way to cool the body. Life and exercise are heating and drying, bathing moistens, and eating and drinking replenish us, but only sleep truly cools us from the action of life. But sleep does more than just cool us. Galen says, "... nothing equally digests everything that can be digested and dispels troublesome fluids as well as sleep after a bath."[337] So sleep is also a great aid to our digestion and to the expelling of our waste. When we suffer from poor digestion or from excessive excrement, we should consider poor sleep as a cause. Hippocrates says: "Want of sleep, after a meal, is injurious, as it prevents the food from dissolving...."[338]

Sleep must be balanced with wakefulness. When sleep and wakefulness are well-balanced, when sleep is about 7-8 hours,[339] it "comforts nature much, refresheth the memory, cheers the spirits, quickens the senses, revives the animal virtue, strengthens the body, helps digestion, and expels

---

336 Anonymous poet quoted in Hygiene, p195.
337 Hygiene, p157.
338 Hippocrates 4, Regimen 2, Ch 60.
339 Culpeper's commentary to Art, Ch 85.

excrements."[340] Too much wakefulness "... makes giddy brains, fills the body full of rheum [excrement], dries the brain, ... troubles the spirits, ... and makes fools,"[341] and too much sleep "... dulls the senses, causes superfluous excrements, makes dull wits, retains excrements, and over-moistens the brain."[342] Basically, lack of sleep overheats the body, and excessive sleep over-cools the body.

The brain must be able to cool down in order to sleep. Many people are chronically "on" in their minds, always thinking, rarely enjoying relaxed mental activity. This makes the brain too hot, and it is simultaneously a result of an overly hot brain. A hot brain feeds off itself. In order to cool the brain, one must learn to enjoy not using one's mind. This is not about vacating one's senses, but about allowing a place for reverie, daydreaming, and art. Reading poetry, slowly and in a relaxed way, can open the door to this kind of cooling of the brain. Even better is *listening* to poetry, listening to music, watching a play, playing with children, swinging on a swing. All things that are passive and that encourage the mind to wander are gateways into reverie, and therefore gateways to cooling a brain that is too hot and too active. Reading a few poems before bed can help those with active minds to cool their brains enough to sleep more easily.

Ensuring that we get enough exercise helps us sleep. Galen says, "... most of those who are engaged in manual labor sleep very heavily, something that contributes greatly to

340 Culpeper's commentary to Art, Ch 85.
341 Culpeper's commentary to Art, Ch 85.
342 Culpeper's commentary to Art, Ch 85.

digestion, they are consequently harmed less by bad food...."[343] As Malidoma Some says, "To truly appreciate sleep one must deserve it. To deserve sleep, one must work hard for it."[344]

Sleep is such an important part of our health regimen that we should all work to ensure that we calm our brains and get enough exercise in order to sleep well. The next chapter on herbs includes information to help balance the brain so that we get better and proper sleep, but in short, the following herbs can help us to sleep better: lettuce, coriander/cilantro, and poppy seeds. Lettuce has the power to help us sleep,[345] simply by including it in our meals we will sleep better. Coriander/cilantro, when eaten last, causes sleep,[346] and poppy seeds are "used to procure rest and sleep...."[347]

Sleeping on a firm surface hardens the body, and sleeping on a soft surface softens the body. These are generalized effects on the entire body, and so can be very imbalancing if used inappropriately. Most people should sleep on a moderately firm surface to avoid generalized softening or hardening of the body.

The healthy time to sleep is at night: "As for the time of sleeping, the day-time is disliked, and the night accounted

---

343 Hygiene, p80-1.
344 Some. *Of Water and the Spirit*. New York: Penguin Group, 1994. P157.
345 Culpeper, p84. Dioscorides, p292.
346 Hippocrates 4, Regimen 2, Ch 54.
347 Culpeper, p125-6.

only fitting."[348] Many people are 'night owls' and prefer to be awake in the night and to sleep through the day, but the tradition of Hippocrates speaks against this practice. The darkness and coolness of the night moves a balanced body toward sleep, and the light and heat of the day rouse it to action. Those who do not follow these patterns are considered imbalanced by Hippocrates and should seek out the root of this imbalance.

If we can remember that sleep is our primary way to cool ourselves, then we will be less likely to discount the need for sleep, making ourselves less likely to find excuses to stay awake when we should be asleep. Without sleep our entire system will easily become imbalanced, becoming too hot, exhausted, filled with excrement, and suffering poor digestion. If we want to be balanced, then we can't skimp on sleep.

---

348 Culpeper's commentary to Art, Ch 85.

Herbs and Remedies for Balance

Up to this point we have mostly assumed that the entire body is equally balanced or imbalanced, but this is not always the case. Each organ in the body has its own balance on its own wobble board. Each organ of the body must be balanced.

It's important that we learn to recognize if, when, and how a particular organ is imbalanced, and that we learn how to balance any imbalances. This chapter will first help us to identify when and how the individual organs are imbalanced, and then it will provide remedies for each organ imbalance.

It is a fortunate person who not only has a reasonably well-balanced constitution, but who also has each and every organ showing the same tendencies toward heat, cold, moisture, and dryness. Most of us have at least one organ that doesn't follow suit with the rest of the body, having, for example, cold and dry lungs in a body that is constitutionally balanced toward heat and moisture. Galen says,

> The constitutions of bodies that are most prone to disease are made up of parts that differ in their temperament, as is the case, for example, with a stomach that is quite hot, but a brain that is cold, and similarly lungs and chest that are sometimes completely cold when the stomach is hot. The reverse often happens when everything else is hotter than

normal and just the stomach is colder, and the same is true for the other parts of the body when the liver is hotter.[349]

We all have our weak spots which are consistently the center of problems: "For many bodies are well-constituted in the head, for example, and poorly in the thorax, the abdomen, and the genitalia. And in some the dyscrasia is in the joints, and in many in some one of the viscera, or in some other one part, or in several...."[350] Most of us will find that we have one or two weak points in our bodies. Some will have a stomach that is susceptible to indigestion. Others will have lungs that are prone to be too dry.

The problem with organ imbalances is that if we attempt to balance them with our usual tools (exercise, massage, bathing, eating, and sleep), then we may end up imbalancing other organs or our overall balance. If we try to balance a cold and dry stomach by eating hot and moist foods for example, we may end up knocking ourselves off the wobble board into a hot and moist disease.

The good news is that certain herbs target certain organs and can help to balance the organs without imbalancing other parts of the body. For example, fennel leaves help to balance a brain that is too hot and moist. Taking fennel leaves does almost nothing to the rest of the body while simultaneously helping to restore balance to a hot and moist brain. Fennel leaves allow us to restore a hot and moist brain to balance even if the rest of the body is cold and dry, an extremely

---

349 Food, p167.
350 Hygiene, p21.

difficult task without such herbs that can target specific organs of the body.

There is a rich tradition of herbal medicine that goes back primarily to the ancient Greek herbalist named Dioscorides. Historian Vivian Nutton says of him: "... Dioscorides and his herbal [became] the bible of medical botany and [exercised] an enormous influence on pharmacology and botany well into the seventeenth century."[351] There is a rich western herbal heritage that goes back through Culpeper in the 1600's to Galen, Dioscorides, and Hippocrates. The last of the great herbalists working in this ancient tradition was Culpeper, whose herbal is heavily referenced in this chapter, and Culpeper's translation of Galen's *The Art of Physick* forms the basis for this entire chapter.

Herbs heat, cool, dry, or moisten specific parts of the body. Different herbs have different strengths, ranging from the first degree, which is the weakest, to the fourth degree which is the strongest. First degree herbs match the healthy human balance, gently leaning us toward balance. They do not push us past the balanced point and so are very safe. Second degree herbs are stronger, helping to restore significant imbalances, but do carry some power to imbalance us. Third and fourth degree herbs have extremely powerful effects which are more proper as medicines than as preventive measures. In this book, we will discuss mostly 1st and 2nd degree herbs, saving the more powerful herbs for those

---

351 Nutton. *Ancient Medicine*. New York: Routledge, 2013. P179.

willing to study much deeper than this book intends to go. By using only 1st and 2nd degree herbs, we keep our herbal remedies relatively safe. But we must always remember that any herb can cause problems and may be severely contraindicated for certain people with certain conditions, especially for those who are taking any form of modern medication. The 3rd and 4th degree herbs, if used without care, can make us sick all on their own. Saffron is a good example. It has wonderful effects, but it can also cause problems. Culpeper explains,

> Saffron is endowed with virtues, for it refreshes the spirits, and is good against fainting-fits, and palpitation of the heart: it strengthens the stomach, helps digestion, cleanses the lungs, and is good in coughs. It is said to open obstructions of the viscera, and is good in hysteric disorders. However, the use of it ought to be moderate and seasonable, for when the dose is too large, it produces a heaviness of the head, and a sleepiness.[352]

As long as we stick to the weaker, more balancing herbs, we shouldn't have problems. Therefore, most of the herbs recommended in this book are 1st degree herbs. They will only restore us to balance. Again, fennel leaves are a good example. They have the power to rebalance a brain that is too hot and too moist, having a cooling and drying effect on the brain, but it is not an extremely strong effect, for it isn't going to make the brain imbalanced toward the cold and dry. First degree herbs just restore balance. Another example is lettuce. It's not so much that lettuce moistens the liver, but

---

352 Culpeper, p144.

that it decreases excessive dryness of the liver. Lettuce brings the liver toward balance, and is a safe food to take as an herb. Of course, eating a pound of lettuce per day may be an imbalancing thing to do for a number of reasons, but eating a small salad each day when the liver seems excessively dry is a balancing thing to do that carries very little risk of imbalancing us.

All of the herbal remedies recommended in this book are easily found at most supermarkets. This is for the ease of the reader and to prove the point that one need not seek out exotic, mysterious herbs to find effective remedies for common problems.

Organs and Their Remedies

The liver is one of the primary drivers of our constitution, so an imbalance of the liver can be devastating to the balance of the entire body. The liver has this power over the entire body because it was imagined by the ancients to generate the blood. An imbalanced liver generates imbalanced blood, and that blood then spreads throughout the entire body. If one is feeling too hot, then the liver may be too hot. Likewise, if one is feeling too cold, then the liver may be too cold. If one is uncomfortable with humid weather, then one's liver may be too moist, and if one is uncomfortable with dry weather, then one's liver may be too dry. In addition, one's overall energy level is a good indicator of the balance of the liver. Hyperactivity is a sign that the liver may be too hot, and lethargy is a sign that the liver may be too cold. One's complexion is also a good sign of the balance of one's liver. A red complexion is a sign of being hot and moist. A yellow complexion is a sign of being hot and dry. A grey complexion is a sign of being cold and dry. And a white complexion is a sign of being cold and moist. The following chart summarizes the general balances of the body:

Balanced	Hot/Moist	Hot/Dry	Cold/Dry	Cold/Moist
Comfortable	Too hot	Too hot	Too cold	Too cold
Comfortable	Too humid	Too dry	Too dry	Too humid
Energetic	Hyperactive	Hyperactive	Lethargic	Lethargic
Radiant	Reddish	Yellowish	Greyish	Pale

Complicating matters is the fact that everything we've so far discussed can also be caused by the balance or imbalance of the heart. The heart is responsible for moving the blood through the body, so it too can cause imbalances throughout the body in much the same way as the liver, and with the same signs. In order to differentiate between the liver and the heart, we can check our veins, which show the balance of the liver, and our pulse, which shows the balance of the heart.

The veins are the easiest way to get a reading on the balance of the liver, with heat making the veins large, cold making them small, dryness making them hard, and moisture making them soft. Looking at the back of one's hands, one will see blueish veins that are usually quite obvious running along the back of the hand. These veins should be noticeable, but not glaringly obvious. If they are not noticeable, as if they don't exist, then they are small veins, which is a sign that the liver is too cold. If they are large and obvious, then the liver is likely too hot. And if they are noticeable but not large, then the liver is probably well-balanced between hot and cold.

One can assess the hardness of the veins by touching them. They should be squishy. If they are so soft that one cannot really feel them, then the liver is likely too moist. If they are hard enough to be easily felt, then the liver is likely too dry. And if they are squishy but noticeable, then the liver is probably well-balanced between moist and dry.

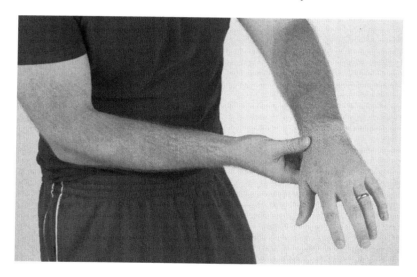

The veins are a subtle thing to assess. It is more useful to look at them on a regular basis for signs of change in the balance of the liver. If the veins are suddenly harder than normal, for example, then the liver is becoming more dry. If the veins are suddenly much smaller, then the liver is becoming colder. The idea of daily assessing the body for changes is key in the thinking of Hippocrates, who recommended watching people closely because the slightest change was a sign of coming disease.[353] If one acted immediately to balance slight imbalances, then health was almost guaranteed. By assessing the veins daily, we can easily notice changes. The following chart summarizes and gives remedies:

Liver Imbalance	Signs	Remedies
Hot and Moist	Large, soft veins	Sweating, diuretic herbs
Hot and Dry	Large, hard veins	Raisins, lettuce, strawberry
Cold and Dry	Small, hard veins	Capers, lettuce, strawberry
Cold and Moist	Small, soft veins	Raisins, cinnamon, fennel, chamomile, sweating, diuretic herbs

An imbalanced liver means imbalanced blood. The blood eliminates excrement through sweat and urine, and so both sweat and urine are important for keeping our blood and liver balanced. Sweating and urinating both cleanse the blood and help to keep it balanced. If the blood becomes too moist, then sweating and urinating are important in order to dry the blood back to balance. People who have moist constitutions and/or moist livers benefit from purposefully sweating and urinating. We can sweat by exercising, bathing, or by taking diaphoretic herbs, and we can urinate by taking diuretic herbs. We've

---

353 Hippocrates 4, Regimen 1, Ch 2.

discussed exercising and bathing in detail in their respective chapters. Now we will discuss diaphoretic and diuretic herbs.

There are two very safe diaphoretic herbs: peppermint[354] and chamomile.[355] A tea made from either one will provoke sweating, but peppermint deserves special attention. It is known to be remarkably safe, short acting, and extremely effective. The herbalist Grieve says, "Peppermint is good to assist in raising heat and inducing perspiration, although its strength is soon exhausted. In slight colds or early indication of disease, a free use of Peppermint tea will, in most cases, effect a cure, an infusion of 1 ounce of the dried herb to a pint of boiling water being employed, taken in wineglassful doses; sugar and milk may be added if desired."[356] These two diaphoretic herbs, peppermint and chamomile, help to balance the liver by removing excess moisture in the blood.

Diuretic herbs work in a similar fashion by removing excess moisture from the blood by provoking urination. There are many diuretic herbs, most of them being foods which we routinely eat. Diuretic foods that we commonly eat include celery,[357] fennel,[358] apple juice,[359] asparagus,[360] kidney

---

354 Grieve.
355 Culpeper, p32.
356 Grieve.
357 Hippocrates 4, Regimen 2, Ch 54. Culpeper, p48.
358 Culpeper, p59. Hippocrates 4, Regimen 2, Ch 54.
359 Hippocrates 4, Regimen 2, Ch 55.
360 Dioscorides, p275. Food, p146.

beans,[361] water cress,[362] pumpkin and squash,[363] spinach,[364] and cucumber.[365] There are a number of herbs that are also diuretic. These include garlic,[366] leek,[367] sage,[368] thyme,[369] oregano,[370] parsley,[371] and chamomile.[372] Whenever we make heavy use of garlic, leek, sage, thyme, oregano, or parsley as seasonings for our food, and whenever we use these herbs and chamomile as herbal medicines, we will see a significant increase in our urine output. These foods help to dry our blood when it is too moist, balancing the liver and the entire body.

Diaphoretic and diuretic herbs both remove excess moisture from the body, thereby balancing the blood, the liver, and the entire body. They are remarkably helpful tools for balancing the body, but we must be careful, for they are only useful for those whose bodies or livers are too moist. Those who are too dry could become severely imbalanced by the use of such herbs.

---

361 Dioscorides, p300.
362 Dioscorides, p283.
363 Dioscorides, p291.
364 Culpeper, p161.
365 Culpeper, p47.
366 Culpeper, p66. Hippocrates 4, Regimen 2, Ch 54.
367 Hippocrates 4, Regimen 2, Ch 54.
368 Culpeper, p147-8.
369 Hippocrates 4, Regimen 2, Ch 54.
370 Culpeper, p88-9.
371 Culpeper, p112.
372 Culpeper, p32.

The liver is very important for our digestion and for our blood. The old way of imagining how the liver functions is that it has tubes connecting it to the intestines through which it absorbs our food and turns it into blood. Obstructions of these tubes cause problems with both our digestion and our blood, giving us a heavy feeling in the bowels and causing the liver to produce imbalanced blood. In the chapter *Eating for Balance* we discussed how appetizers and the proper ordering of a meal can prevent the liver from getting obstructed, but there are also herbs which can help. These include celery,[373] parsley,[374] bay leaves,[375] rosemary,[376] and thyme.[377] Of thyme, Culpeper says: "Use garden-thyme in all your drinks and broths, it will prevent stoppages [of the liver] before they come, and cure them after they are come."[378] Ensuring that the liver stays unobstructed is good insurance for keeping the entire body balanced, and regular use of these herbs can do just that.

The heart is the other major driver of our overall balance. The heart can be assessed by the pulse and by our breathing. The hotter the heart, the faster it beats, so a hot heart will have a fast pulse. A cold heart does not necessarily slow the heart below its normal resting rate, so instead we have to rely on a low energy level and the sense of being too cold to give us a sign that the heart is too cold. In much the same way as

---

373 Culpeper, p48.
374 Culpeper, p112.
375 Culpeper, p13-14.
376 Culpeper, p138.
377 Culpeper, Last Legacies #49.
378 Culpeper, Last Legacies #49.

the liver affects the hardness of the veins, the heart affects the hardness of the pulse. When the heart is too moist, it has a soft pulse, and when it is too dry, it has a hard pulse. By taking the pulse at the wrist we can assess the balance of the heart. This is especially valuable as a sign for change in the balance of the heart. By taking one's pulse on a daily basis, changes can easily be identified. A faster pulse means the heart is becoming hotter, a slower pulse means the heart is becoming colder, a softer pulse means it is becoming more moist, and a harder pulse means it is becoming more dry.

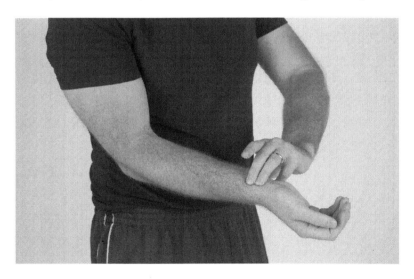

There are equivalent changes in one's breathing that should match with one's pulse. A heart that is too hot makes one breathe fast, a moist heart makes one breathe deeply, and a dry heart makes one's breathing shallow. The ancient way of imagining the function of the lungs was that by taking in air from outside, they kept the heart from overheating. Their function was to ensure that the heart did not get too hot.

When we are active and the heart must work hard, the lungs breathe faster to cool the heart.

When assessing the veins, pulse, and breathing, it's best to do so at the same moment in the day, since each of these signs will change depending on one's activity and position. A great time to assess the veins, pulse, and breathing is first thing in the morning or at the end of one's warm-up for exercise, which is when the veins, pulse, and breathing should all be relatively consistent from day to day.

To summarize, a hot and moist heart will have a fast, soft pulse causing one to breathe fast and deep. A hot and dry heart will have a fast, hard pulse causing one to breathe fast and shallow. A cold and dry heart will have a hard pulse causing one to breathe shallow. And a cold and dry heart will have a soft pulse causing one to breathe deeply. The following chart summarizes the heart imbalances and gives the remedies:

Heart Imbalance	Signs	Remedies
Hot and Moist	Fast, soft pulse and fast, deep breathing	Sweating, lemon juice, lemon seeds
Hot and Dry	Fast, hard pulse and fast, shallow breathing	Lettuce
Cold and Dry	Hard pulse and shallow breathing	Saffron
Cold and Moist	Soft pulse and deep breathing	Exercise, nutmeg, cinnamon, saffron, rosemary

Since the function of the lungs is so intimately connected to the function of the heart, these two organs affect each other's balance. Maintaining the lungs in a balanced state is important for maintaining the heart in a balanced state, which in turn is important for maintaining the balance of the entire body. Lungs that are too hot spill their heat over to the heart because they cannot keep the heart cool. There are no symptoms commonly associated with hot lungs, so a heart that is too hot may be the only sign of hot lungs. Hot lungs can easily become dry lungs because the heat burns up all their moisture. Likewise, cold lungs are susceptible to becoming too moist. Cold lungs are able to do their job well to keep the heart cool, but they become sensitive to breathing cold air and to becoming too moist.

One sure sign of a lung imbalance is a cough. The lungs purge themselves of excrements primarily by coughing.[379] So coughing is a sign of having excessive excrements in the lungs. A dry cough is a sign of dryness in the lungs; a wet cough a sign of moisture in the lungs. When the lungs are too dry, one's voice becomes rough and raspy, and when the lungs are too moist, the voice becomes muddy. Dry lungs also make one thirsty with an unquenchable thirst. Drinking liquids does nothing to satisfy one's thirst when the lungs are the cause of the thirst. Lungs can become too moist because of excessive excrement flowing down from the head. We will discuss this in detail shortly, but for now, it's important to recognize that the head may be the ultimate cause of excessively moist lungs. The following chart summarizes lung imbalances and remedies that we can use.

Lung Imbalance	Signs	Remedies
Hot	Hot heart signs	Cool the heart
Cold	Sensitivity to cold air	Almonds, figs, dates, raisins
Moist	Muddy voice, wet cough	Purge and dry the head
Dry	Unquenchable thirst, raspy voice, dry cough	Poppy seeds

---

379 Art, Ch 99.

Thyme is a remarkable herb because it has great benefits and is almost completely harmless.[380] It helps to balance the lungs no matter what their imbalance, and so is a good herb to use whenever a lung imbalance is suspected.

Having a cough is a sure sign that the lungs are imbalanced in some way, full of excess excrement. Sage tea is helpful for hoarseness and coughs,[381] and oregano helps coughs.[382] Both of these herbs can be used to help alleviate coughing. In addition, nuts can be very helpful for clearing the lungs. Galen says: "All nuts that contain a sufficient amount of that overpoweringly bitter quality [almonds, in particular] are extremely useful for the spitting up of matter and of thick and viscous moisture from the lungs and chest."[383]

The brain affects how we think and sleep, two crucial aspects of life and balance. A brain that is too hot makes our minds wild and frantic, making us erratic and likely to make poor decisions. A hot brain has great difficulty calming down enough to go to sleep, and when it does get to sleep, it has wild and disturbing dreams. On the other hand, a cold brain is slow and muddy. It makes thinking unclear and decisions poor. A cold brain is already halfway asleep, and it would prefer to slump off into dreamland all day. A well-balanced brain, being neither too hot nor too cold, is engaged and active (but not frantic) when awake, and gets refreshed from easy sleep at night.

---

380 Culpeper, p183-4.
381 Culpeper, p147-8.
382 Culpeper, p88-9.
383 Food, p132.

A good indicator of the balance of one's brain is one's eyes. Red, bloodshot eyes are a sign of excessive heat, and runny, tearing eyes are a sign of excessive moisture. Excessive moisture also causes dullness of the senses, making vision, hearing, smell, and taste less clear.

The brain purges its excrements primarily through the mucus in the nose which is expelled by sneezing.[384] A regular assessment of this mucus, which was called rheum by the ancients and which is commonly known as snot, is a good indicator of the balance of the brain. If there is copious amounts of rheum, then the brain is probably excessively moist, and if there is no rheum at all, then the brain is probably too dry. The following chart summarizes the imbalances and remedies for the brain:

---

384 Art, Ch 99.

Brain Imbalance	Signs	Remedies
Hot and Moist	Feeling rushed, lots of excrement in the head, dull senses, disturbed sleep	Fennel leaves
Hot and Dry	Feeling rushed, little excrement in the head, disturbed sleep	Lettuce
Cold and Dry	Feeling slow, little exrement in the head, excessive sleep	Strong beer/wine with sugar and nutmeg, sage
Cold and Moist	Feeling slow, lots of excrement in the head, dull senses, excessive sleep	Chamomile, fennel, oregano

Keeping the brain and head balanced is of great importance for the rest of the body because the head drains into the rest of the body. The excrement in the head, when not adequately expelled, drains down from the head into the lungs and stomach via the throat and causes imbalances in these organs,[385] which in turn can imbalance the rest of the body. So if the excrements in the head become excessive, the rest of the body can become imbalanced. For this reason it is important to keep the head clear by keeping the excrements

---

385 Hygiene, p262-3.

in the head thin and easily purged. The excrements are purged first through the nostrils, second through the mouth, third the ears, fourth the hair, and fifth the eyes. It is the nostrils that are the most proper and fitting way to purge the head, and this is done by sneezing. A daily practice of clearing the nose by blowing it and sneezing is important for the health not only of the head but of the entire body. Mucus flowing down the back of the throat, what is called post-nasal drip, is a sign that we are not clearing the excrements of our heads through the most appropriate means: the nose.

Many problems are caused by the head not being purged. Galen says,

> ... it is obvious ... that uvulitis, and tonsillitis, and gingivitis, and cervical adenitis, and dental caries, and ulcers and pyorrhea in the mouth, are due to the catarrhal ichors descending to them from the head. ... the great majority of doctors either incise the uvula or give drugs to promote expectoration of what has flowed down through the trachea into the lung. But some treat the stomach, some the teeth and mouth, or even the conditions in the nose. Let me omit the eyes and ears, although their lesions are not a few. For it were better, I think, to remove the source of the trouble by strengthening the head....[386]

And Culpeper concurs, saying:

> Whosoever would keep their mouth, or tongue, or nose, or eyes, or ears, or teeth, from pain or infirmities, let them often use sneezing, and such gargarisms [gargling with certain herbs]; for, indeed, most of the infirmities, if not all, which

---

386 Hygiene, p260.

infest those parts, proceed from rheum [excessive excrement from the head].[387]

Many common problems, including dental decay, indigestion, chronic coughs, and ear infections, are due to not keeping the head clear of rheum. In order to keep our head clear of excessive excrements, remedies that induce sneezing, clear the nasal passages, and thin the mucus in the head are all helpful.[388] Culpeper recommends gargling to purge the head, saying, "The head is purged by gargarisms [gargling with certain herbs], of which mustard… is excellent...."[389] Garling is a singular aide for purging the head because it allows us to use strong herbs that may otherwise imbalance us without actually taking them internally. Mustard is a great example. Seasoning our food with mustard is great for clearing the head, but it has a powerful heating effect. If the body and/or head are also cold, then eating mustard is helpful and balancing, but if the head and body are already too hot, then mustard will further imbalance the head and/or body even while purging the head of excrements. It may purge excrements, but it will simultaneously create an excess of new ones by imbalancing the head and/or body. By gargling with mustard, we thin the rheum without heating the head and body at the same time. Gargling allows us to use an herb and then spit it out so that it doesn't affect the balance of our entire body.

---

387 Culpeper, Last Legacies, #22.
388 Hygiene, p269.
389 Culpeper, Last Legacies, #2.

For those who are too hot and who need to clear their head of rheum, Galen recommends taking prolonged baths of fresh water, allowing the warm vapors to dispel the excrement in the head.[390] Hippocrates recommends walking first thing in the morning to dry the head and to thin the rheum for easier purging,[391] and Galen says that obstructions of the head can be cleared by walking before and after meals.[392] All of these are excellent things to do to keep the head clear.

In addition there are a number of herbs that can be used to help purge the head of rheum. Rosemary helps to expel rheum especially in a head that is too cold.[393] Dioscorides says that the smell of basil causes sneezing which can help to clear the nasal passages.[394] Three more-drastic measures involve snuffing herbs up one's nose. Onion juice,[395] dried, powdered oregano,[396] and dried, powdered cayenne pepper have all been used for this purpose. To snuff some herb up one's nose, one simply takes a very small amount of the herb, barely enough to notice it on the hand, and then sniffs it up the nostrils. It is wiser to keep the rheum from ever becoming such a problem that one would snuff something up one's nose to expel it, but sometimes these more drastic measures may be appropriate. Perhaps the most gentle and useful of ways to prevent and expel excessive rheum in the head is to

---

390 Hygiene, p263.
391 Hippocrates 4, Regimen 2, Ch 62.
392 Hygiene, p254.
393 Culpeper, p138.
394 Dioscorides, p296.
395 Culpeper, p109.
396 Culpeper, p88-9.

chew sage.[397] Chewing sage thins and helps to remove the rheum.

But we shouldn't think that the head and brain alone are all we need to consider to keep the head clear. The other organs are also vitally important. Culpeper says: "... be sure, if you would keep your brain clear, keep your stomach clean."[398] All the organs interrelate and affect each other, so they're all important. But the stomach and brain have a unique relationship. Excess excrement in the head flows down and causes imbalances in the stomach, and disturbances in the stomach cause vapors to rise out of the stomach up to the head and cause imbalances in the head.[399] We need to keep them both clear if we want to be healthy.

But we don't want to over-complicate matters. As much as the head can cause stomach problems, Culpeper makes it clear when he says that "Infirmities of the stomach usually proceed from surfeiting [eating excessively]."[400] The stomach, although it can be weak and easily imbalanced, is usually troubled from overeating. Whenever we suffer stomach problems, we should first look to the obvious cause and ensure that we haven't been gorging ourselves.

The stomach is the key to our digestion. If it doesn't function well, then the entire body cannot properly replenish itself. Problems in the stomach directly affect the head, liver, and

---

397 Culpeper, p147-8.
398 Culpeper, Last Legacies, #22.
399 Hygiene, p262-3.
400 Culpeper, Last Legacies #42.

bowels, and from the liver affect the balance of the blood and therefore the entire body. One of the keys to health is to keep the stomach well-balanced. A well-balanced stomach has a large appetite and doesn't have strong cravings for extremely moist foods (soggy and slimy) or extremely dry foods (such as burnt toast). A small appetite is a sign of a cold stomach. Cravings for moist foods means the stomach is too moist, and cravings for dry foods means the stomach is too dry. In addition, a dry stomach makes one thirsty and yet drinking liquids causes digestive upset (belching). Indigestion is the clearest sign of stomach imbalance. An excessively hot stomach causes greasy belching, and an excessively cold stomach causes bloatedness and flatulence. The following chart summarizes its imbalances and the remedies for each imbalance:

Stomach Imbalance	Signs	Remedies
Hot	Indigestion with greasy belching	Strawberry, lettuce, barley, cucumber
Cold	Indigestion with bloating and flatulence	Ginger, fennel, mint, sage, nutmeg, cinnamon, pepper, rosemary, oregano
Moist	Lack of thirst and craving moist foods	Cinnamon, mint, sage, rosemary, nutmeg, anise seeds, pepper
Dry	Thirsty but cannot tolerate liquids, craving dry foods	Lettuce, apples, cherries, strawberries, oranges, lemons, cucumbers, prunes

The safest bet to help a disturbed stomach is to take oxymel, which is a combination of honey and vinegar. It cuts thick juices in the stomach without heating or cooling the stomach, and therefore is very helpful to the stomach without risking imbalancing the stomach.[401] Whenever we have excess rheum flowing down the back of our throats, it's a good idea to take oxymel as a preventive measure to help keep the

---

401 Hygiene, p264.

stomach strong. The following is a recipe for oxymel: 1) boil honey, skimming and discarding any foam that forms on top; 2) add apple cider vinegar (half as much as the honey that was used) and boil again so that the honey and vinegar are thoroughly mixed and the vinegar is cooked; 3) set this away for storage; 4) when ready to use, mix one part oxymel in two parts water, and then drink.[402] The proportions of this recipe are very flexible. Galen says, "... it is better to judge the proportion by the patient's own sensations... considering that the pleasantest oxymel is most suitable for the patient's nature, and therefore also beneficial...."[403] More or less honey, vinegar, or water is perfectly acceptable. It should be an enjoyable thing to drink.

If the stomach shows signs of being too cold, then we can add pepper and cinnamon to oxymel to help to heat the stomach in addition to strengthening it. Or we can try another of Galen's recipes, a concoction that both strengthens and heats the stomach: 1) mix two pints apple juice, two pints honey, and one-and-a-half pints vinegar; 2) simmer gently, skimming and discarding any foam that forms; 3) mix in three ounces of ginger and two ounces of pepper, and simmer again until it is the consistency of honey.[404]

Another thing that we can do for the stomach is to gently massage the abdomen.[405] The pressure of a massage helps to keep the stomach and bowels functioning well, and it is

---

402 Hygiene, p165.
403 Hygiene, p165.
404 Food, p201, Note 5.
405 Hygiene, p263.

very helpful especially as a preventive measure when other factors, such as excess excrement in the head, may interfere with the function of the stomach. But we should only massage the abdomen when the stomach is empty. A full belly doesn't take kindly to massage.

A common irritation of the stomach is heartburn. It can be caused by either a cold or a hot stomach, and should be balanced according to the remedies above, but the symptoms themselves can also be alleviated. Hippocrates recommends coriander (also known as cilantro) for this purpose.[406] Adding coriander/cilantro as a seasoning to one's meal can help when one is plagued by heartburn.

A major sign of imbalance in the body is loss of appetite, and this is often caused by a weak and cold stomach. Oregano restores the appetite,[407] bringing the stomach back to its proper function. Oregano is mildly warming, so it is a fairly safe herb, but it can overheat an already hot stomach, so it must be used wisely.

Imbalance of the bowels is a common problem and one that Hippocrates believed to be of paramount importance.[408] When the bowels get imbalanced, we must immediately take action to bring them back to balance because imbalanced bowels will imbalance the entire body and cause illness. Balancing the bowels involves a change in exercise, diet, massage,

---

406 Hippocrates 4, Regimen 2, Ch 54.
407 Culpeper, p88-9.
408 Hippocrates 4, Regimen, Book 3, Ch 79-82.

bathing, and sleep. There are no simple herbal remedies for bowel imbalances.

Our bowel movements tell the story of our bowels.[409] They should be easy and, though not necessarily smelling sweet, they should not be remarkably stinky. Properly digested food does not smell all that bad, and bowels that are working well have bowel movements that come out solid but without effort. Watery stool is a sign that the bowels are too moist, and dry stool is a sign that the bowels are too dry. Undigested, stinky stool is a sign that the bowels are too cold. The following chart provides a summary of each type of bowel imbalance and what remedies are appropriate:

---

409 Art, Ch 99.

Bowel Imbalance	Signs	Remedies
Hot and Moist	Watery but digested stools	Less exercise, walking, tepid baths, less food, cool and dry foods[410]
Hot and Dry	Dry, constipated stools, and dry, bitter mouth	Less exercise, short amounts of gentle exercise, bathe daily, get enough sleep, cool and moist foods[411]
Cold and Dry	Undigested stools	More exercise, vigorous and swift exercise, walking, morning massage, oil the body daily, warm baths, lots of sleep, less food, moistening foods[412]
Cold and Moist	Watery, undigested stools	More exercise, vigorous and swift exercise, walking, lots of massage, avoid bathing, eat less, drying foods[413]

---

410 Hippocrates 4, Regimen 3, Ch 81.
411 Hippocrates 4, Regimen 3, Ch 82.
412 Hippocrates 4, Regimen 3, Ch 80.

Balancing the imbalances of the bowels is a taller order than balancing the imbalances of other organs. Simple herbal remedies will not do the trick. It requires a change in one's entire regimen to rebalance the bowels. For this reason, one should take care to maintain a healthy balance of the bowels.

Certain foods can help to purge the bowels of excess excrement and help to keep them balanced. Hippocrates says: "Juices that send to stool or purge are those of chickpea, lentils, barley, beet, cabbage...."[414] We can eat these foods to help to keep our bowels clean.

Each tissue of the body, the joints, muscles, tendons, and sinews, can become imbalanced. It's important to recognize when a tissue becomes imbalanced and to take action to remedy the situation. When a tissue is too hot, it will feel warm to the touch and often suffer from a sharp pain. Cold tissues will feel cold to the touch, be slow to warm-up, often moving in an uncoordinated manner, and are usually stiff. Soft tissues are either too moist or excessively relaxed. They will feel soft to the touch and will often be larger than normal. Hard tissues are either too dry or excessively tensed. They will feel hard to the touch and will often look smaller than usual. A great time to assess all the tissues of the body is during the preparatory massage and movements for a workout. We touch and move everything during this time, giving us a great opportunity to assess any imbalances. One

---

413 Hippocrates 4, Regimen 3, Ch 79.
414 Hippocrates 4, Regimen 2, Ch 54.

thing of which we must be aware is the possibility of a general imbalance affecting many of our tissues at once. For example, if a couple of tissues all appear to be hot and soft at the same time, then it is likely that each of those tissues have become imbalanced on their own, but if many tissues suddenly appear to be hotter and softer than usual, then it is likely that the body in general has become imbalanced toward the hot and moist. In a general imbalance, remedies for the individual tissues will prove almost worthless; instead the remedy should be aimed at the general balance of the body. On the other hand, when an individual tissue is imbalanced, a specific remedy to the tissue will prove most effective. The following chart summarizes the imbalances of tissues and provides remedies for each imbalance:

Tissue Imbalance	Signs	Remedies
Hot	Tissue is warm to touch, sharp pain	Less exercise of the region, cool bath with chamomile
Cold	Tissue is cold to touch and doesn't warm-up easily, stiffness	Longer warm-up of the region , massage with oil, warm bath with sage, rosemary, and/or oregano
Soft	Tissue is soft to touch	Longer, more vigorous exercise of the region; long, firm massage of the region; uncomfortably cold bath
Hard	Tissue is hard to touch	Shorter, less vigorous exercise of the region; short, gentle massage; long comfortable bath with chamomile and oregano

The tissues of the body are greatly affected by exercise, massage, and bathing. Each of these topics have been discussed in detail in their respective chapters, but we have not yet discussed bathing in water that is infused with certain herbs. Herbs placed in a bath can affect the tissues of the body. Chamomile, sage, rosemary, and oregano are the four herbs we will discuss.

Bathing in chamomile removes fatigue and takes away irritation from the body. It helps strained sinews, and it only slightly warms, so it is safe for tissues that are too hot. Chamomile has the reputation of helping all pains.[415] It is one of the truly blessed herbs.

Any form of joint or sinew pain can be alleviated by sage. It can be eaten, placed over the painful tissues, or placed in one's bath water.[416] Bathing in sage, rosemary, and/or oregano warms cold tissues, and so bathing in these herbs is best used when the tissues are cold.[417] Oregano also softens hard tissues, so it is particularly helpful to bathe in oregano when tissues have been hardened.[418]

The above discussion of each major organ and its imbalances should help us all identify if and when an organ is imbalanced and how we can remedy the situation.

---

415 Culpeper, p32.
416 Culpeper, p147-8.
417 Culpeper, p138, 147-8.
418 Culpeper, p88-9.

Specific Herb Discussion

There are a number of commonly-used herbs that deserve special discussion. Garlic is one such herb. It is a powerful but dangerous herb. Culpeper says it is very useful:

> ...being a remedy for all diseases and hurts (except those which itself breeds).... Its heat is very vehement, and all vehement hot things send up but ill-favored vapours to the brain. In [hot and dry] men it will add fuel to the fire; in men oppressed by [cold and dryness], it will attenuate the humours, and send up strong fancies, and as many strange visions to the head: therefore let it be taken inwardly with great moderation and outwardly you may make more bold with it.[419]

Since garlic is such a powerful herb, we should feel free to use it gently as a seasoning in our food, letting our taste be our guide, but we should be careful not to make immoderate use of it, and we should not use it as an herb unless we are sure it will be safe for us. It can powerfully cut excessive cold and moisture from the body and purge the head of rheum, but it also heats the brain and can cause severe imbalance. Onion is very similar to garlic, and almost as dangerous.[420]

Cayenne pepper is similar to both garlic and onion in its powerful and potentially dangerous effects on the body.[421] It is excellent for eliminating phlegm from the body, cutting it and helping it to move more easily. It's especially helpful as a seasoning for meats so that they do not cause us to take in

---

419 Culpeper, p66.
420 Culpeper, p109.
421 Culpeper, p127.

too much thick nourishment that will fill us with phlegm. But because it is so powerful, it can imbalance us very easily. Instead of using it as an herbal remedy, we should simply use it as a seasoning and allow our taste to guide us.

Mustard is yet another powerful herb with which we must be careful.[422] Culpeper says of it: "[Mustard] is an excellent sauce [seasoning]... for weak stomachs... but naught for [hot and dry] people, though as good for such as are aged, or troubled with cold diseases."[423] Just as for garlic, onion, and cayenne pepper, mustard is best used as a seasoning because it has potentially dangerous powers when used as an herb. However, mustard has one very important remedy for which we can use it safely, and that is as a gargle as we discussed earlier. By spitting it out, it doesn't affect the entire body, but just purges the head. It can also be rubbed on the nostrils, forehead, and temples to induce sneezing to help purge the head,[424] and should then be washed off immediately.

There are a few herbs that are on the opposite end of the safety spectrum from the dangerous garlic, onion, cayenne, and mustard. These herbs are so gentle, safe, and harmless that one would need to be significantly imbalanced for any of them to cause any problems. These gentle herbs include chamomile, thyme, celery, parsley, and peppermint.

---

422 Culpeper, p96-7.
423 Culpeper, p96-7.
424 Culpeper, p96-7.

Chamomile is a gentle and safe herb, being only slightly warming.[425] It helps all pains,[426] which is a remarkable power, and it helps digest what needs digesting,[427] that is, it helps us digest our food and it helps to expel all excrements from the body. This is one of the truly great herbs.

Culpeper specifically tells us that thyme is very harmless.[428] The wonderfully helpful powers of thyme have been listed throughout this chapter, and it is nice to know that it is also an extremely safe herb to take.

Likewise, celery is said to be suitable to all constitutions because it has the power to cool while simultaneously opening the body.[429] There are few people who wouldn't benefit from including this mild, safe, but effective herb in their diet. The same is true of parsley, which does essentially nothing bad while enhancing the flavor and appearance of food, soothing the stomach, and calming and preventing flatulence.[430]

Along with chamomile, thyme, celery, and parsley, peppermint has a reputation of being very harmless. We've discussed its use as a diaphoretic earlier. There is one other very useful power of mint, and that is its ability to make milk easier to digest. Culpeper says, "[Mint] suffereth not milk to

---

425 Culpeper, p32.
426 Culpeper, p32.
427 Culpeper, p32.
428 Culpeper, p183-4.
429 Culpeper, p48.
430 Culpeper, p112.

curdle in the stomach, if the leaves thereof be steeped or boiled in it before you drink it: Briefly, it is very profitable for the stomach."[431]

The ancient way of imagining the body included a number of problematic fluids. Two fluids in particular need constant monitoring and evacuation, and those are bile and phlegm. Bile is hot and dry; phlegm cold and moist. Being too hot and/or too dry, eating hot and dry foods, and having a hot and/or a dry constitution can cause a buildup of bile in the body, making one prone to be hectic and angry, and making inflammatory pains common throughout the body. Being too cold and/or too moist, eating cold and moist foods or even too much food, and having a cold and/or a moist constitution can cause a buildup of phlegm in the body, making one prone to being lethargic and to having difficulty removing excrement from the body. Those who are hot and moist and those who are cold and dry are prone to both excesses of bile and phlegm. Those who are hot and dry have a harder time with bile, and those who are cold and moist have more difficulty with phlegm.

Whenever either of these fluids becomes excessive in our bodies, we become easily imbalanced. It's important to expel them regularly. Certain herbs can help to evacuate these problematic fluids from the body. Hippocrates specifically mentions oregano for its ability to evacuate bile.[432] Whenever we are plagued by hot and dry imbalances, we would be wise

---

431 Culpeper, p94.
432 Hippocrates 4, Regimen 2, Ch 54. Culpeper, p88-9.

to add oregano to our food in order to help expel any bile building up in our bodies.

Phlegm is a constant problem for almost everyone, but especially during the cold and moist time of the year. There are a number of herbs that help to expel phlegm from the body. These include thyme,[433] fennel,[434] bay leaves,[435] garlic, onion, and cayenne. We've discussed the dangers of garlic, onion, and cayenne, so these three herbs should be used for this purpose only in extreme cases. But thyme, fennel, and bay leaves are relatively harmless and can be used regularly to not only expel phlegm but to prevent it from becoming excessive.

There are a few other common and mild herbs that have specific and useful effects worthy of discussion. Strawberry, for instance, quenches thirst.[436] It is a very useful food to eat when one is thirsty to prevent the need to drink excessive amounts of liquid. Strawberries also cool the blood.[437] This can be an extremely helpful power for those who are too hot and for during the hot times of the year.

Cucumber juice helps to cool the eyes.[438] Placing a slice of cucumber over one's closed eyes is an excellent way to

---

433 Culpeper, p183-4. Hippocrates 4, Regimen 2, Ch 54.
434 Culpeper, p59.
435 Culpeper, p13-14.
436 Culpeper, p173.
437 Culpeper, p173.
438 Culpeper, p47.

soothe eyes that are red and irritated from a brain that is too hot.

Oregano helps itches and scabs.[439] Eating oregano or placing it over an irritated part of the skin can both help the skin.

Rosemary warms and helps all cold imbalances of all the organs.[440] Even though it is not listed as a useful remedy for each organ, rosemary helps all organs rebalance against cold. For this reason it can be a very useful remedy for those who have a cold constitution, for everyone during the cold months of the year, and for anyone suffering from multiple organs that are imbalanced toward cold.

The herbal remedies in this chapter are a wonderful and incredibly useful tradition on which we can draw. They can benefit all of us by helping to keep each organ balanced. For any reader who wants to learn more about herbal remedies and wants to draw upon the ancient tradition of Western herbal medicine, both Culpeper's *English Physician* and Dioscorides' herbal are worthy reads.

---

439 Culpeper, p88-9.
440 Culpeper, p138.

What Would Hippocrates Say?

Now that we have covered each tool at our disposal for balancing ourselves on the wobble board of health (exercise, massage, bathing, eating, sleeping, and herbs), it is time to see it all from the big picture. This chapter attempts to succinctly answer the question: what would Hippocrates say? We will cover a number of common issues, including the basic imbalances, being too hot or too cold, too moist or too dry, and also how to lost fat, gain muscle, balance old age, and handle a busy or a lazy day.

When well-balanced we desire what is balancing, but when imbalanced we desire what will further imbalance us, and so health often requires us to work against what we are inclined to do, to exercise when we would like to rest, and to rest when we would like to be active, to eat meat when we don't have an appetite for it, and to abstain from meat when it sizzles with delectability. A simple example to which we can all relate is exercise in cold versus hot weather. When the weather is warm, our bodies are warm and ready for action and exercise comes more easily, but we need much less exercise when the weather is warm than we do when it is cold. And when the weather is cold, our bodies are cold, making it much harder to get ourselves moving, decreasing our desire to engage in exercise. But this is exactly when exercise is most beneficial. For balance, we cannot just trust our desires. In fact, balance often requires us to work directly against our desires. A perfectly balanced specimen should exercise, massage, bathe, eat, and sleep so as not to disturb the balance. That is, exercise and massage should be moderate, food should be balanced neutrally so as not to warm, cool, dry, or moisten, and bathing and sleep should be taken in moderation.[441]

As we work through these various ways to balance under certain circumstances, remember that health abhors sudden change, so even if one is severely imbalanced toward too much heat and moisture, for example, and it turns out that one isn't following a very cooling and drying regimen, one shouldn't jump full force into a cooling and drying regimen. A slow, calm approach is always wisest. We should always make slow changes to our regimen.[442]

The following tables summarize the regimens most appropriate for the primary imbalances.

---

441 Hygiene, Book 2, Ch 12.
442 Hippocrates 4, Aphorisms, Book 2, Ch 51.

Too Hot and Too Moist

Signs
Hyperactivity, feeling too warm and humid, sweaty, and disturbed sleep.

Exercise
Take lots of slow exercise, such as walking.

Massage
Infrequently take long massages to purge the body.

Bathing
Take short cool or cold baths or showers. Occasionally take long baths to purge excrement.

Eating
Avoid overeating.
Take one meal per day.
Thin Foods: cool and dry foods such as asparagus, artichoke, lemons, limes, oranges, apples, pears.
Thick Foods: cooler and drier thick foods such as fish and millet.
Minimize fat in your diet, using olive oil instead of butter when you do use fat.
Minimize sweeteners in your diet, using raw honey when you do use a sweetener.
Drink water with lemon, peppermint tea, and chamomile tea.

Sleep
Ensure that you get enough sleep.

Remedies
Check your liver and heart for excessive heat and moisture. Sweating and diuretics.

Too Hot and Too Dry

Signs
Hyperactivity, feeling too warm and dry, parched, chapped, and disturbed sleep.
Exercise
Take little, if any, exercise, and emphasize slow exercises such as walking and weightlifting.
Massage
Infrequently take moderate duration massages.
Bathing
Take long, cool baths.
Eating
Avoid undereating.
Take two meals per day.
Thin Foods: cool and moist foods such as lettuce, plums, strawberries, melons, cucumbers, and sour grapes.
Thick Foods: cooler and moister thick foods such as barley and boiled fish and chicken.
Minimize fat in your diet, using butter instead of olive oil when you do use fat.
Minimize sweeteners in your diet, avoiding raw honey when you do use a sweetener.
Drink water and water with cucumber.
Sleep
Ensure that you get enough sleep.

Too Cold and Too Dry

Signs
Lethargy, feeling too cold and dry, parched, chapped, sleeping excessively.

Exercise
Take a short amount of exercise emphasizing swift exercises such as running.

Massage
Frequently take moderate duration massages.

Bathing
Take long, warm baths.

Eating
Avoid undereating.

Take two meals per day.

Thin Foods: hot and moist thin foods such as figs, sweet grapes, winter squash, carrots, radishes.

Thick Foods: hot and moist thick foods such as meat, milk, and butter.

Use butter instead of olive oil when you use fat.

Drink warm liquids, tea, and red wine.

Sleep
Ensure that you aren't sleeping excessively.

Too Cold and Too Moist

Signs
Lethargy, feeling too cold and humid, sweaty, sleeping excessively.

Exercise
Take lots of exercise emphasizing swift exercise such as running.

Massage
Frequently take long massages to purge.

Bathing
Take short, warm or hot baths. Occasionally take long baths to purge excrement.

Eating
Avoid overeating.

Take one meal per day.

Thin Foods: hot and dry thin foods such as cabbage, beets, onions, garlic.

Thick Foods: hot and dry thick foods such as fish and wheat.

Use olive oil instead of butter when you use fat.

Use raw honey when you use a sweetener.

Drink warm liquids, tea, and wine.

Sleep
Ensure that you aren't sleeping excessively.

Balancing Fat and Muscle

Hippocrates and Galen have excellent ideas for fat loss:

> Fat people who wish to become thin should always fast when they undertake exertion [exercise], and take their food while they are panting and before they have cooled, drinking beforehand diluted wine that is not very cold. Their meats should be seasoned with sesame, sweet spices, and things of that sort. Let them also be rich. For so the appetite will be satisfied with a minimum. They should take only one full meal a day, refrain from bathing, lie on a hard bed, and walk lightly clad as much as is possible. Thin people who wish to become fat should do the opposite of these things, and in particular they should never undertake exertion when fasting.[443]

Seasoning food with satisfying, sweet spices and making them rich and thick makes them satiating, stopping us from eating excessive amounts of them. Taking only one meal per day is thinning. Not bathing and sleeping on a hard surface both toughen the body, hardening it. Walking is the key exercise in Hippocrates' view, allowing us to get lots of exercise without risking much injury.

To this, Galen adds that swift exercises and abundant thin nourishment are the keys to removing excess fat.[444] Swift exercise melts the flesh more than any other form of exercise and so is very helpful for fat loss. And by eating lots of thin nourishment, one becomes full and satiated without eating excessive amounts of thick nourishment, allowing the body to

---

443 Hippocrates 4, Regimen in Health, Ch 4.
444 Hygiene, p257.

easily lose body fat. Combining this with what Hippocrates says, if one wants to lose fat then one should do lots of walking, some fast running, eat small amounts of rich thick nourishment, but emphasize large amounts of thin nourishment.

Culpeper adds fennel to the list, saying: "Both leaves, seeds, and roots [of fennel], are much used in drink or broth, to make people lean that are too fat."[445] So fennel is an excellent choice of thin nourishment to help with fat loss. And Galen also says that gentle massage, too little or too slow of exercises, too much sleep, and poor digestion can all cause fat gain.[446] So if we want to lose fat, then we must ensure that we get the rest of our regimen in order also.

It's important to understand that Hippocrates doesn't make a blanket statement that everyone needs to lose fat. On the contrary, Hippocrates and Galen both discuss strategies for gaining mass along with strategies for losing fat because it was considered just as unhealthy to be too thin as it was to be too fat. Remember, moderation is key. A moderate amount of fat is healthy, and neither thinness nor fatness is healthy. This is really one of the major signs of the wisdom of the ancients. They recognized that excess in any direction was unhealthy. In the modern world, we talk about the obesity epidemic in our country, but there is also an almost unrecognized epidemic of leanness. Many people are so concerned about being fat that they have gone to the other

---

445 Culpeper, p59.
446 Hygiene, p192.

extreme, and it's killing them faster than the fat would have killed them. Being fat at least helps keep one moist, staving off the effects of the dryness of old age. Being skinny drys the body way too quickly. The point is that one should strive to find the happy medium, the sweet spot of being neither fat nor thin. For most of us, this is a large, easily-attainable plateau.

Hippocrates has a clear strategy for weight gain. He tells us to do just the opposite of what we'd do to lose fat, and in particular he emphasizes that if we want to gain mass then we should never exercise when fasting.[447] Galen recommends that we seek out the reason for why we are too thin. The causes he lists include: working or thinking excessively, taking too much swift exercise, taking too much massage or bathing, not sleeping enough, being excessively hot, not drinking enough, and not eating enough.[448] He also says that leanness is often caused by weak digestion.[449] Galen recommends three ways to help a body to increase in size and weight:[450] the first is a moderate amount of exercise, the second is a moderate duration of massage to encourage blood to flow into the flesh to help it grow, and the third is oiling the body, which moistens the body to help it grow. In addition, the great herbalist Dioscorides says that cheese is good for weight gain.[451] The following charts help to show how to adjust one's regimen for these purposes.

---

447 Hippocrates 4, Regimen in Health, Ch 4.
448 Hygiene, p192.
449 Hygiene, Ch 6, 8.
450 Hygiene, p25.
451 Dioscorides, p209.

How to Lose Fat

Exercise

Take lots of exercise, specifically lots of walking and swift runs. De-emphasize slow exercises such as weightlifting. Fast when exercising.

Massage

Avoid gentle massage.

Bathing

Avoid bathing.

Eating

Eat while still warm from exercise. Eat lots of thin nourishment (especially fennel) and small amounts of rich and satisfying thick nourishment. For example, have multiple courses of vegetables followed by a small portion of a favorite meat dish. Drink warm liquids. Eat one meal per day.

Sleep

Sleep on a hard surface and ensure that you aren't sleeping excessively.

How to Gain Mass

Exercise
Ensure that you aren't exercising too much or using too much swift exercise. A moderate amount of slow exercise such as weightlifting helps to build the body. Never exercise on an empty stomach.

Massage
Ensure that you aren't taking too frequent or too long of massages, but oil the body daily.

Bathing
Ensure that you aren't bathing too frequently or for too long.

Eating
Ensure that you aren't under-eating. Cheese is particularly helpful. Ensure that you are drinking enough liquids.

Sleep
Ensure that you are getting enough sleep.

Balancing Old Age

One thing we are all heading toward is old age, which is a cooling and a drying of the body. No matter how hot and moist we are, we are always slowly growing colder and drier. For this reason, we should all know what to expect and how to balance against the effects of age.

Old age is primarily due to drying.[452] Galen says we get drier as we age, and this is certainly true. But at extreme old age moisture begins to return to the body as it decays into death. This is the winter season of life, where so much of the heat of life has dissipated that moisture begins to accumulate within the body because there is no sufficient means of expelling it. The seasons of life go from the moist heat of childhood, to the dry heat of adulthood, to the dry cold of old age, to the moist cold of extreme old age.[453] But practically speaking, dryness is the enemy that brings us into old age.

Both bile (hot and dry) and phlegm (cold and moist) accumulate in older bodies because the coldness attracts phlegm and the dryness attracts bile. So older people must take care to routinely purge excrements to ensure that they do not get overwhelmed by them. Galen says: "... because... excrements collect in the body of old men, it is necessary to provoke urination daily, not with drugs, but with barley and honey and with diuretic wines, and to move the bowels,

---

452 Hygiene, p7.
453 Hippocrates 4, Regimen 1, Ch 33.

mostly with oil, administering it before meals."[454] Everything we've discussed in this book about excreting excrements should be routinely and gently used in old age. This includes sweating through gentle exercise, infrequent long massages, long warm baths, adequate amounts of sleep, and diuretic and diaphoretic herbs.

As for exercise, Hippocrates says, "No old man needs complete quiescent [rest], nor violent exercise."[455] The older we get, the more we should focus on exercises to which we are accustomed, giving up the intense forms of them.[456] Exercise should be routinely practiced, but never close to causing injury. The extremes are even more unwise in old age. Moderate exercise is the absolute rule for the aged.

Older people should focus their exercise on their strengths.[457] If, for example, an older person has naturally strong legs and is more prone to injury in the arms, then he or she should make primary use of exercises for the legs, allowing the arms to be strengthened indirectly. If, for example, an older person is naturally inclined toward endurance activities instead of strength activities, then he or she should focus on endurance activities and allow them to slightly add strength to the body. By following their strengths, the aged can take more exercise with less risk of injury. This allows them to exercise regularly in order to keep the body warm. The young can work to

---

454 Hygiene, p216.
455 Quoted by Galen in Hygiene, p195.
456 Hygiene, p195.
457 Hygiene, p195.

balance their weaknesses, but the old should give up such aims.[458]

Hippocrates has an interesting saying about the injuries and illnesses of older people. He says: "Old men generally have less illness than young men, but such complaints as become chronic in old men generally last until death."[459] Young people with their hotter and moister nature end up with more acute problems, but these problems come and go easily enough. The colder and drier nature of older people keeps things cooler and thus less likely to explode, but when things do happen, they last for a long time. So it's very important for older people to prevent injuries because these injuries will last much longer.

Frequent, short massage is helpful to warm and moisten an aging body. A morning massage is a great way to help keep the body moving well.[460] In addition, warm baths are also helpful to both warm and moisten the body. Long baths can be very helpful to purge excrement while moistening and warming.[461]

Drinking wine (which is warming) instead of water (which is cooling), and eating warm and moistening foods is very helpful in old age.[462] Fasting is easier the older one is[463]

---

458 Hygiene, p195.
459 Hippocrates 4, Aphorisms, Book 2, Ch 39.
460 Hygiene, p195.
461 Hygiene, p195.
462 Hygiene, p195.
463 Hippocrates 4, Aphorisms, Book 1, Ch 13-14.

because with less of the flame of life burning in one's body, there is less flesh melted each day and therefore less need and desire to replenish oneself. But this doesn't mean that older people should fast. On the contrary, Galen recommends that older people eat more frequently than younger people. Three meals per day was his general guideline for the aged. The first meal should be very light, perhaps just bread with honey, and the last meal intentionally kept small to prevent indigestion, which becomes more common with old age.[464]

Galen's *Art of Physick* includes a succinct prescription for the aged:

"The healthful causes which amend [old age] are such things which give present and secure nourishment... they consist in moderate motion, meat, drink, and sleep. As for motion, ... walking, and rubbing themselves are convenient, after which, let them cool, and ease themselves by degrees. As for meats, let them first take such as are moist and easy of digestion (but let them avoid cold meats as much as may be) afterward let them eat such as are of good nourishment; for drink, let them drink good wine, and now and then a cup of wine after meat...."[465]

This simple advice can help many an aged body. The following chart illustrates a regimen for old age.

---

464 Hygiene, Book 5, Ch 4.
465 Art, Ch 100.

Balancing Old Age

Exercise
Take daily, gentle exercise of short duration with an emphasis on sweating to purge the body.

Massage
Take frequent, short massage to warm the body, especially in the morning, and take infrequent long massage to purge the body.

Bathing
Take long, warm baths to warm, moisten, and purge the body.

Eating
Eat multiple times per day, ensuring that you do not cause indigestion from taking too large of meals, especially in the evening. Emphasize heating and moistening foods and warm liquids.

Sleep
Ensure that you are getting enough sleep.

Balancing the Physicality of the Day

If we aren't going to exercise on a given day, then we will want to heat, dry, and harden our bodies in some other way. Our massage should be longer and harder. Our bath should be warmer and shorter. Our food should be warmer and drier. And we should ensure that we don't take too much sleep. Exercise expels excrements, and so if we aren't going to exercise, we'll need to expel excrements in other ways. This can be through a long massage, a long bath (which is only balancing for those who are too dry), or with diaphoretic and diuretic herbs.

At the other extreme, if we have a physically, emotionally, and/or mentally challenging day, such as helping a friend move, digging up a stump, starting a new job, giving a major presentation at work, or attending a funeral, then we must recognize the 'exercise' that we've already taken for the day. Life itself is heating and drying, and a particularly challenging day of life is very heating and drying. We should take less or even no exercise on such days. Performing just apotherapy and massage may be our best bet for the day. Galen says: "... after wakefulness, or grief, or both, let [exercise] be the apotherapeutic."[466] A cooler bath is in order. Cooler and moister foods are wise. And more sleep is almost a necessity.

---

466 Hygiene, p135.

Balancing a Non-Strenuous Day

Exercise
Try to fit a walk into the day.
Massage
Take a harder and longer massage.
Bathing
Take a long, warm bath.
Eating
Eat less food.
Sleep
Ensure that you are getting enough sleep.

Balancing a Strenuous Day

Exercise
Try to fit a walk or apotherapy into the day.
Massage
Take a shorter massage.
Bathing
Take a long bath, adjusting the temperature to balance how you feel.
Eating
Eat less food.
Sleep
Ensure you get enough sleep.

Gentle Cleansing Purge

Waste accumulates in the weak parts of the body because the stronger parts of the body can push the waste away and so eventually the waste settles in the weakest parts of the body. Therefore treatment for an organ that periodically hurts, especially if it follows a seasonal pattern, getting worse during certain times of the year and better at others, is to reduce the diet and purge the body. This is especially true in springtime: "Such as are benefited by... purging shall be purged... in spring."[467] If such a cleansing purge removes the discomfort and leaves us vibrant, then it is a useful technique. But we must take care, for such a cleansing purge can make us too dry and too thin, and it can be very damaging to purge the body excessively and leave it imbalanced toward dryness and thinness.[468]

People who are too hot and too moist are too full of blood. Excess blood fills the body, making it likely to incur both fatigue and injuries. Tension Fatigue can occur even without exercise because the excess blood makes tension inside the tissues of the body, and injuries can occur very easily because hot blood can easily cause tissues to overheat.[469] Nosebleeds are common during these times because nosebleeds are a spontaneous way of removing blood from the body.[470] Hot and moist times were the classic time to

---

467 Hippocrates 4, Aphorisms, Book 6, Ch 47.
468 Hygiene, Book 6, Ch 13.
469 Hygiene, p178.
470 Hygiene, p179.

'bleed' a patient by puncturing an artery and draining blood out of the body. (This cannot be recommended in this modern age, and would only be performed by a trained physician in ancient times.) But there are other ways to reduce the blood. Sweating is a powerful way to decrease excessive hot and moist blood, as is taking exercise and using diaphoretic and diuretic herbs. Being too moist means that excessive excrement is likely to build up in the body. Purging the blood by ensuring that excrement is removed from the body through exercise, bathing, defecation, and urination is the key to rebalancing.[471] Bathing after exercise and before meals is recommended for everyone, but it is particularly recommended for those who are hot and moist to help purge excrements.[472]

To perform a cleansing purge, we avoid all violent activity, at the most taking a walk for exercise, gently massaging the body with oil, taking mild baths, resting without food, and sleeping as much as possible.[473] This simple technique can work well to purge the body of excess excrements. It's essentially a short fast lasting about 16 to 20 hours accompanied by rest and relaxation.

---

471 Hygiene, p245.
472 Hygiene, Book 6, Ch 3.
473 Hygiene, p157.

One-Day Cleansing Purge

This simple, one-day cleanse is useful as a springtime purge, when seasonal symptoms appear, such as allergies and skin irritations, and for those who are too moist.

Exercise
Take the day off from exercise, avoiding all violent activity and all forms of strenuous work, including physical, emotional, and mental. Short, easy walks are helpful.
Massage
Take a long massage to purge excrement from the body.
Bathing
Take a long, warm bath to purge excrement from the body.
Eating
Eat no food during the day and take only small amounts of liquids.
Sleep
Take plenty of sleep, napping during the day if possible.

The Voice of Health

In this chapter we're going to explore how what Hippocrates says has to do with our vitality. Health is a very important aspect of vitality. It's hard to imagine having a sense of vitality without also feeling healthy, comfortable in one's skin, lacking aches and pains, suffering from no digestive upsets.

Longevity is another aspect of vitality, the sense of living a long, fruitful life. We've said a number of times how the key to staying healthy, especially as we age, is to prevent the drying of the body: "... he who dries the least will live the longest."[474] But Heraclitus, the most ancient of philosophers speaking at the beginning of Western thought, says: "Dry, the soul grows wise and good,"[475] and he isn't alone in speaking well of dryness. In cultures throughout history, an elder is revered for his or her age, recognized as a dry, wise soul. Dryness relieves one of moisture, one's youthful attachment to the unnecessary aspects of life, even to life itself. Dryness initiates one into the wisdom of death. In the tradition of astrology, one begins life ruled by the closest 'planet' to the earth, the Moon, which is the planet of moisture, and ends life ruled by the farthest visible planet, Saturn, the dry planet. Dryness may not be healthy, but it certainly is wise.

---

474 Hygiene, Book 6, Ch 3, p244.
475 Haxton. *Fragments*. New York: Penguin Group, 2001.
  #74.

By trying to prevent drying, Hippocrates can be understood to be an enemy of old age and of wisdom, an enemy of death. And an enemy of death is an enemy of life, for it denies the reality that all life ends in death. Galen even goes so far as to say that decrepit people are better off dead.[476] The attitude of health is an attitude that denies the legitimacy of living with pain and suffering. Death is understood to be better than an imbalanced life.

In order to be balanced, one must curb one's desires, for "Hot bodies desire hot nourishment, cold bodies cold nourishment, dry bodies dry nourishment, and moist bodies moist nourishment, and the reason is because every like is maintained by his like."[477] So when we are imbalanced, we crave the things that will keep us imbalanced and that will make us even more imbalanced! We must restrain our desires in order to be healthy. We need to really hear what Hippocrates says: to be healthy, we cannot live how we desire! In fact, we must live exactly how we don't desire, eating hot foods when we desire cold, and cold ones when we desire hot. Those who follow their desires are specifically derided by Hippocrates: "[There are those who live] just as they please, and would neither forgo nor restrict the satisfaction of any of their desires."[478]

But the poet William Blake says: "Those who restrain desire, do so because theirs is weak enough to be restrained."[479]

---

476 Hygiene, Book 5, Ch 1.
477 Art, Ch 86.
478 Hippocrates 1, Ancient Medicine, Ch 5.
479 Blake, The Marriage of Heaven and Hell.

Imagine a life in which one never follows one's desires: Never eating a slice of chocolate cake! Those who desire to lift heavy weights, the people who truly love the feeling of ripping a ton of weight off the ground, are usually the same people who really don't need to lift heavy weights, who are actually being imbalanced by such activity. Those who enjoy long runs are the people who really need to stop running if they are to be balanced and healthy. Those who just want to relax on the couch and watch television are the people who most need to get out and exercise. Those who want meat need vegetables, and those who want vegetables need meat. A life lived in balance is a life lived without satisfaction. It could be argued that it's not even really a life lived at all: a life lived in balance is a life wasted.

The voice of health says to adjust back to mid-line, to never allow anything to go anywhere: "... [the] chief concern [is] to make no innovation so long as the body is completely healthy, but whenever there is any shift away from the correct balance, immediately to introduce whatever is missing, before the deviation from the state of nature becomes a large one."[480]

We need to be really aware of the effects of listening to the voice of health, for the voice of health is the voice of mediocrity. Galen says, "... whatsoever is immoderate one way, must be brought to mediocrity by its contrary

---

480 Selected. P68.

immoderate...."[481] All things must be taken captive to mediocrity.[482] Health is mediocre! A healthy life is mediocre.

Mediocrity is perhaps nowhere less desired than in the field of athletics, for athletics is about the pursuit of excellence, the drive for victory, for achievement far surpassing mediocrity. The ancient Greeks had the word *arete*, roughly translated as 'excellence,' to explain the pursuit of athletic perfection. There is perhaps no greater opposition than that of *arete* and the balanced health of Hippocrates. Hippocrates tells athletes to train hard in the winter, but in the summer to only walk in the cool of the morning and evening.[483] This severely limits the athlete's skills. There is no way to truly excel at one's sport when following the voice of Hippocrates. Health makes mediocre athletes.

Health does not progress. It is a balance. A cycle is a great image for health because a cycle also doesn't progress. It keeps heading towards where it has already been. So for health it is totally reasonable to work hard to get strong by lifting weights for six months and then to essentially stop, allow fitness to regress, and then start again the following year, each year attaining a fair amount of strength, but never getting beyond that. This non-progressive attitude of health is opposed to the progressive attitude of excellence, which is the athletic drive for victory. We must sense the difference between balanced health and that of victory, which is more associated with the peak performance that we think of when

---

481 Art, Ch 89.
482 A play on St Paul from 2nd Corinthians 10:5.
483 Hippocrates 4, Regimen of Health, Ch 7.

we think of athletics. The perfection of Hippocrates is a perfect, calm balance, while the perfection of athletics is a stretched-to-the-limit, barely maintainable reach toward victory.

The voice of Hippocrates is a balancing, normalizing force. He sees a weakness and wants to strengthen it. He sees an excess and wants to diminish it. 'All things in moderation,' he says. But think of what this really means. If one is a naturally talented runner, then Hippocrates would advise one to not run much and to instead focus on weightlifting. If one is a naturally talented discus thrower, Hippocrates would have one focus on running instead. If one is naturally inclined to activity, having a hot constitution, Hippocrates would have one rest more. And if one is inclined to spend one's day relaxing, Hippocrates would get one out to exercise. Hippocrates would make us balanced and normal. He would make us all the same. He would make life square. Instead of playing to our strengths, he would have us ignore them. Hippocrates would stop us from developing our talents, and he would stop us from following our desires. The big, natural football players would be at home with their books, and the football field would be crowded with skinny guys who would prefer to be reading. The voice of health can prove to be the death of talent and enjoyment, the death of vitality. So, what would Hippocrates say? Who cares!? If his plan is to curtail our strengths and make us 'normal,' then all he'll do is end up ruining our lives!

But let's be fair. Hippocrates doesn't want to ruin our lives, he just wants to make sure that our lives don't end prematurely, and that we don't spend our lives suffering needlessly from diseases that are completely preventable. What it boils down to is that Hippocrates has great advice for us, but his advice must always be taken with an ear for its destructive tendencies. If he succeeds in helping us live long and healthy lives but simultaneously makes us dull and boring, devitalizing our lives, then he isn't worth following. If instead we live lives brimming with vitality, playing to our strengths and to our desires and to our pleasures, and he can help us not die too young and not be too riddled with diseases, then he will have served his role well.

We are a very health-obsessed society, and so it is hard for us to hear the difference between health and vitality. We usually equate the two words in our minds. But health is the desire for lack of disease, the desire for comfort, and vitality is the drive to live life to the fullest. The reality is that vitality asks us to run a marathon, eat a slice of pie, and stay up all night watching a great movie or having fun with friends or getting drunk, while health tells us to jog a quarter mile, eat steamed carrots, and go to bed early. Health and vitality are wildly different things. They are often diametrically opposed. Vitality can make us decidedly unhealthy, and health can kill vitality.

Honestly, who wants to live an extra (even healthy) ten years if those ten years aren't spent doing and enjoying the things one loves? Who wants to eat flat, flavorless 'health' food for the rest of one's life? Who wants to never stay up late at night to enjoy an evening with friends just because it hinders one's healthy sleep? Who wants to never smoke a cigar (if one enjoys them) just because it is bad for one's health? Life is simply too short to make health a top priority! Of course, there's a flip side to all this. For who wants to live if one is sick all the time, suffering aches and pains, and coughing up phlegm from too many puffs on the cigar? Of course, health and vitality are both important. Vitality shouldn't be allowed to completely destroy one's health, but even more important, health shouldn't be allowed to destroy one's vitality, which is the trap in which so many people get caught in this modern world. Most of us are either caught by an obsession over health, or have abandoned all pretense of health, favoring complete debauchery over the ridiculously devitalizing rules of the 'healthy.' Both of these extremes are the result of an imagination that takes the idea of health way too literally. Health must be a part of vitality, not the other way around. The key is how we imagine both health and vitality. Instead of trying to force vitality within the limited confines of health, we need to find a way to fit health within vitality.

Let's take bathing for example. People with a hot constitution shouldn't take hot baths or sit in a jacuzzi, but people with hot constitutions generally love to steep themselves in near-boiling water for prolonged periods of time. To ask them to stay away from hot water is to ask them to make their lives significantly less delightful. And then to tell them to take cold showers instead is about as horrific of an idea as one can possibly devise. It's torture!

Eating the way Hippocrates tells us to eat is perhaps the most dangerous thing that is recommended in this book. For Hippocrates treats food as medicine, and nothing can be more destructive to a life of vitality than the eating of nothing but medicine, of eating food for the sake of one's health rather than for the sake of one's appetite, tastes, and desires. Eating food may be the most enjoyable experience of life. It is certainly one of the best things we do. Many people call it orgasmic. Hippocrates and his 'healthy' ideas make food into medicine and meals into balancing acts. It's perfectly fine to eat a 'healthy' meal by incorporating steamed vegetables in order to help balance excessive dryness, but one must insist upon its deliciousness. Buy only the highest quality seasonal vegetables, steam them to perfection, and season them delectably. Demand taste!

Health is one form of vitality, but only *one* form. There are many other types of vitality, most of which are decidedly unbalanced.

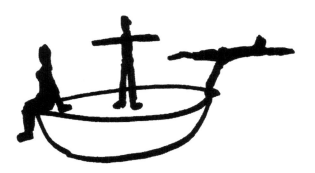

The image above illustrates three different aspects of vitality. In the center is the safe, balanced poise of health. On the right is the image of an athlete reaching to the absolute limit and almost falling. On the left is a relaxed person in passive reverie allowing life to float by, which is deceptively dangerous by hanging off the edge, far from balance. All three of these, and many more, are legitimate forms of vitality that all play a role in our lives.

Along with mediocrity comes a blindness to beauty that is inherent in the pursuit of balanced health. For example, there is a pace at which the body wants to run. This pace will be different for everyone, but it certainly exists. Hippocrates would tell us to run at a balancing pace, that is, at the pace that will make one pant when the balancing distance has been covered. Hippocrates doesn't care for the pace at which the body *desires* to run. But suppose we were to ask Marsilio Ficino, the Renaissance physician whose translations of certain ancient works of Plato were the rebirth of many ancient ideas that were of prime importance to the movement of the Renaissance. What would Ficino say? He would have us run at the body's *desired* pace and for as long as the body desires. He would have us run for the pleasure of it, otherwise not at all.

Similarly, there is a rhythm and a speed at which each body wants to walk. It is the comfortable, pleasurable pace. Each body is different, but, when conversing with another person, a collective pace and rhythm establishes itself. These are unconscious things that occur when people are just going about the business of life. It is these natural rhythms that Ficino would have us follow. He would have us walk without a thought to how fast we are walking. Hippocrates, on the other hand, prescribes the pace and distance depending on one's imbalances. For Hippocrates, balance is paramount. For Ficino, beauty, desire, and pleasure are paramount.

While on the topic of walking, Ficino prescribes a daily walk for exercise. But not just any walk will do. He tells us to walk in a beautiful garden, exercising the soul in the beauty, not simply the mechanical motions of the body. For Ficino, the body and soul are completely tied together: what is good for one must also be good for the other. Comparing this to Hippocrates, we find no parallel. To Hippocrates, a walk on a treadmill inside an air conditioned gym while watching television would have a similar effect as walking outdoors. In fact, if one is in need of cooling and drying, the air conditioning may even prove more balancing than walking outdoors in a beautiful garden. The lack of a demand for beauty in life becomes apparent in the voice of Hippocrates. We would all be well-advised to ask 'What would Ficino say?' after asking what Hippocrates would say, otherwise our balanced life may end up an ugly one. All of this is to continue to make the point that the voice of health can be a destructive voice, even an ugly voice, in our lives. We do not want to follow Hippocrates blindly.

Compared to Ficino, what Hippocrates has to say can seem rather soulless. Imagining how we can heat, cool, moisten, or dry the body, replenishing what is lost and depleting what is in excess: the ideas of Hippocrates take measure of the body and attempt to balance the measures. For Hippocrates, the body is somewhat of a machine. The way that Hippocrates imagines the body is the starting point for the modern separation of body and soul, what has led to the body being imagined purely in mechanical terms. But although Hippocrates may be the start of the mechanical imagination, he is far from it. The body and soul are still deeply united within his thinking. His ideas, measuring the body not by the modern objective measures of chemicals, x-rays, and functional questionnaires, but in the images of heat, coldness, dryness, and moisture (which correspond to the four elements of fire, water, earth, and air), maintains an amazingly living image of the body. Historian Vivian Nutton describes the living body of Galen's imagination:

> The liver was responsible for nutrition. In the liver 'digested' or 'concocted' food received from the stomach and intestines was turned into nutritious blood, which was then transported within veins to provide the essential nutriment for all the body. Every living being, plants as well as animals, was provided by the Creator with the four 'natural faculties' of attraction, assimilation, excretion and growth. Each part of the body had thus the potentiality, as a result of its elemental organization, to feed on the nutritious blood, to assimilate whatever it needed to grow and function, and to excrete potentially harmful residues that it no longer needed. The body was a living universe, responding to changes and actively seeking whatever it needed in order to exist and to function. Galen's vitalist approach thus contrasted with the mechanistic understanding of the body proposed by [his rivals], in which, for instance, the excretion of residues through the kidney and bladder did not require any active participation from the

organs themselves but only obedience to the laws of physics.[484]

In Galen we find expressed the fantasy of a body that is vitally alive and full of power, the body as imagined in the tradition of Plato, as opposed to the modern view of the body as a machine. By following the line from Culpeper back to Galen back to Hippocrates, we root our fantasy of health in the fantasy of a living body that flows with vitality, a little model of the cosmos that radiates beauty and is full of soul, and we avoid the dehumanizing and soul-destroying notions of the body as a machine.

So although the voice of health is the same voice that turns the body into a machine, that measures its every subtle change, and that eventually separates the body from the mind and soul, the ancient voice of health, the voice of Hippocrates, allows us to imagine health within a still vitally alive body. Hippocrates is a way to escape the modern mechanical imagination while still listening to the voice of balance and health. Hippocrates allows us to work toward health without making the body into a machine. Hippocrates stands at the threshold between the modern mechanical view of the body and the ancient vitally-alive view of the body. He can help us to live in both worlds.

This brings us to the crux. The voice of Hippocrates, jabbering moderating, balanced, mediocre health advice in our ears, is an immensely important voice of vitality that can

484 Nutton. *Ancient Medicine*. New York: Routledge, 2013. P239.

serve us extremely well. The voice of Hippocrates can serve as a voice of healthy vitality in our lives, making room in an otherwise vitally alive life to still attempt some semblance of balance and comfort. If we can imagine Hippocrates as our personal health adviser, then his image can take on a powerful role in our lives. He can shake his head 'no,' reminding us that certain foods will really imbalance us. He can scream at us to stop running, or to start running, when it would be balancing to do so.

By imagining him as an adviser, we can ignore him or reject his advice whenever we would like to do so. But he keeps us honest. He can say, "That slice of chocolate cake will imbalance you," but we can eat it anyway. We can hear him and then decide how important eating this slice of cake really is. He can say again, "That second slice of chocolate cake is really going to imbalance you!" And again, we can ignore him, but we're less likely to ignore him when we've already ignored him once before. By imaging him as an adviser, he becomes a helpful, though often annoying, voice that we can choose to follow or ignore.

In this way, the voice of Hippocrates becomes a servant of vitality. Health itself becomes a servant of vitality. Instead of running our lives and inhibiting all of our decisions, making life mediocre, the voice of health helps us to only do the crazy things that really make our lives more wonderful, and it helps us to feel good and be healthy while we live our lives.

The words and ideas of this book should be imagined as the voice of a benevolent adviser who tends to us daily. Each day

Hippocrates examines us and the effects of the world and makes recommendations for our health. But he is not a taskmaster. He is an adviser.

How does what Hippocrates would say fit into our vitality? We can imagine what Hippocrates says as a wonderfully useful way to take care of the body, to keep it functioning well, and to make us comfortable. It is the vitality of comfort that is perhaps most at play. By exercising, massaging, bathing, eating, and sleeping the way Hippocrates would tell us to do, we make our bodies feel good. We keep away many aches and pains that result from excessive or deficient exercise. We rarely suffer colds and indigestion. We sleep well at night. The ideas of Hippocrates shared in this book are effective ways to feel good. We have here ancient wisdom, developed over centuries, about how to help our bodies to be comfortable. Of course, comfort isn't all that exciting, or tasty. It doesn't lead to victory or championships. In fact, it specifically keeps us from these things. And so comfort can destroy our lives by destroying our vitality. But sometimes comfort is exactly what we desire, and it is at these times that the voice of Hippocrates is most vitalizing.

This book provides us a default health regimen. We should fall back on simple exercises that never hurt us, balanced meals, and good sleep. But when the call of vitality comes, we follow it. If winning the championship is truly worth the sacrifice, if going to war is necessary, if it's Thanksgiving feasting, if it's one's anniversary, then live!: up all night with one's spouse, bloated and jolly (and drunk), injured from excessive training, wearied, bloody, and battle-scarred. There is a way through this conundrum of health and vitality. All we have to do is ask Hippocrates. Everyday we need to ask ourselves: "What would Hippocrates say?" By asking, we keep health imaginative, and prevent it from becoming the concrete shackles that it has become for so many of us in the modern world.

It's hard to imagine the idea of vitality without a significant overlap with the idea of health. It's hard to imagine having vitality and not having health, unable to do much more than sit on the couch because of arthritic hips, coughing fits from diseased lungs, weak limbs, fat bellies, being filled with melancholy or having a bitter demeanor. These don't seem like images full of vitality, for they are so far from the image of health. And yet, the pursuit of health is one of the most dangerous pursuits because it can so easily hinder other forms of vitality. Health is the form of vitality that gives us a sense of balance, of comfort in our lives, of the absence of being uneasy, and the actual creation of ease. The word 'ease' means 'elbow room.' Health gives us room to live our lives. So we want to pursue health and yet not allow it to spoil our vitality. We want to pursue health in a way that enhances our vitality. It cannot become an obsession. We want health to support and empower vitality. And that's just what asking "What would Hippocrates say?" does.

We want the advice of Hippocrates not so that we can be perfect or live longer, but so that he can help to keep us reasonably balanced while we live lives that are not all that reasonably balanced, so that we can follow our desires in life without being sick and uncomfortable all the time, so that we can enjoy the heat of the summer without wanting to punch everyone around us, and so that we can enjoy the cold of winter without being stiff all day long.

Conclusion: The Fantasy of Health

A major question still haunts this book, lurking through its pages: will these ideas actually make us healthier by today's standards? The answer is yes. Since these ideas are all about moderation in all things, these ideas are certainly good for improving and maintaining health. If we follow the ideas in this book, then we'll exercise, but not too much, we'll eat, but not too much, we'll be able to live life without excess or deficit. We will live healthy, comfortable lives if we follow the ideas of Hippocrates. What this book is really about is moderation. The ancient ideas of Hippocrates give us a way to imagine what moderation is. Instead of an amorphous concept, we now have the image of balancing on a wobble board, keeping ourselves from getting too hot, cold, dry, or moist. We have all sorts of ways to imagine what pushes and pulls us in the various directions, and how we can lean in each direction in order to maintain our balance. And we have the image of Hippocrates as our personal health adviser. Hippocrates helps us to reimagine health as balance, and balance as moderation in all things.

The reality is that we would rather *feel* healthy than *be* healthy. Our fantasy of health is to sleep without indigestion, to wake up feeling refreshed, to get out of bed without any part of our bodies aching, to defecate with comfort, to eat wonderful meals without feeling bloated, to exercise not only without pain but to feel great during and after it, to have energy for life, to have energy for sex, to smell good naturally, to have nice breath, to not suffer during life. This is a very important point. The vitality of health is the *subjective* experience of health, and it is what we really crave. It is not the literal definition of health, which can actually kill our vitality, for which we should strive. For example, if health can partly be defined by fitness, and if fitness can be defined as strength, endurance, and mobility, then we can literally improve our strength by lifting weights, which will literally improve our fitness and thus literally improve our health. But lifting weights might easily exhaust us and injure us, leaving us not only literally less healthy, but, more importantly, feeling less healthy, enjoying life less, and having less vitality. The literal idea of health is not really what we want. We want the *feeling* of health, for the feeling of health is a major aspect of vitality. It is the sense of being balanced. The ancient ideas, which we all know to be literally and scientifically false, can be remarkably effective at helping us achieve the imaginary balance that we seek, because this ancient way of imagining health keeps things at the imaginary level.

Literal longevity has absolutely nothing to do with vitality. No one really cares how long they live. They care about how *well* they live. No one really cares about their blood pressure, they care about not having a heart attack. So to live life trying to be 'healthy' in order to prevent disease and in order to sustain life is to waste one's life. But to go out of one's way in order to feel good on a particular day and in order to wake up refreshed, not bloated or fatigued, is certainly a wonderful thing to do. The vitality of longevity comes from connecting to the roots of one's life, to one's ancestors; to deeply sense how one's life is a continuation of the life of one's parents, grandparents, and deep into the dawn of humanity; and to deeply yearn for the continuance of one's life into future generations, which need not be a literal continuation through one's literal children, but can also include one's character influencing the lives of other people, spreading one's soul into the world. This is expressed wonderfully by Walt Whitman:

> What is commonest, cheapest, nearest, easiest, is Me,
> Me going in for my chances, spending for vast returns,
> Adorning myself to bestow myself on the first that
>   will take me,
> Not asking the sky to come down to my good will,
> Scattering it freely forever.[485]

What we are after then in this book is a poetic sense of health and longevity, a subjective feeling of well-being, a comfortable existence of balance, an imaginary sense of health instead of a literal, provable, objective, measurable, concrete and ultimately useless reality of health.

Let's not get lost in an argument about what is healthy. The most important thing to get from this book is the recognition of the voice of health. The voice of health may not be saying what Hippocrates says. Perhaps a gluten-free diet is the voice of health in one's life, or a vegan diet, or a consistent weightlifting program, or jogging five miles per day. Perhaps

---

485 From Song of Myself #14 by Walt Whitman.

the voice of health is saying not to smoke, to get more sleep, to drink less coffee, to drink more coffee, to drink tea instead of coffee, to walk more. There are many ways that the voice of health can speak to us, and many things it might say. In this book, we are trying to hear the ancient voice of health, the voice of Hippocrates, because it helps us to not take health too literally, and it also helps us to rely on ancient principles instead of the latest fly-by-night fads. The desire for health is easily caught in the fads of the moment. The image of Hippocrates helps us to avoid such things. It grounds us in a 2500-year tradition.

A brief discussion of two current health fads is appropriate. The first is the scientifically-supported idea that a diet high in vegetables and fiber is good for one's health. Looking at this from the perspective of Hippocrates can be very illuminating. Vegetables and fiber are thin nourishment. They thin the body and balance against excessive thick nourishment and lack of exercise. For a person who eats lots of meat and doesn't get enough exercise, Hippocrates would agree that a diet high in vegetables and fiber would be balancing and healthful. But Hippocrates wouldn't agree that this sort of diet would be healthful for everyone at all times. A thin diet would be imbalancing for someone who exercises a lot and who doesn't eat much thick nourishment such as meat. The ancient view is here much wiser than the modern view of blanket-statements that are thought to apply to everyone. Likewise, the second modern fad is the idea that lots of exercise, especially cardiovascular exercise, is healthy. This is again true from the perspective of Hippocrates if a person is excessively moist or fat, but it is not true for someone who is excessively dry or thin. In both of these instances, the modern view is dogmatic and simplistic, while the voice of Hippocrates rings true.

The real message of this book can be summarized in two sentences. The first is: one should do all things in moderation unless it would make one vitally alive to do otherwise, in which case one should be extraordinarily immoderate. And the second sentence is: by asking "what would Hippocrates say?" we can more readily know what moderation is. The words of Hippocrates and Galen carry hundreds of years of traditional knowledge on how to perfect moderation, but that's really all they're saying: if health is the aim, then be moderate.

Let's get real about how wise and advanced these ancient people were. Hippocrates, writing near the dawn of Western thinking, knew that diet and exercise were the keys to health. Diet and exercise only became popular and important recently, over the last 50 years or so, in our modern world. The ancients were advocating for diet and exercise 2500 years ago. We are far behind them. By the time Galen was writing in the second century, there was already more than 500 years of work with diet and exercise. Instead of listening to these ancient ideas with a grain of salt, we should be attentively hanging on every word they have to say. Most ancient health advice with which modern thinking currently disagrees will probably turn out to be correct.

Let's hear that last sentence for the fantasy that it carries: ancient wisdom is wiser than modern knowledge. This is the fantasy that was at work in the Renaissance, as historian Vivian Nutton describes:

> When, in the medical Renaissance of the fifteenth and the early sixteenth centuries, the writings of the ancient Greeks were rediscovered by humanist scholars and read again in their original Greek in Western Europe for the first time for a thousand years, the belief was widespread that, through this return to the very springs of medicine, the accretions of later error and uncertainty could be purged away.[486]

The same fantasy can be said to be operating in this book as was operating back in the Renaissance, that of the fantasy of returning to the beginnings in order to get a fresh start, to be reborn, and to discover the true root from which we can all flourish. This book chases the fantasy of health to its ancient roots, invoking the fantasy of the Renaissance, a rebirth of health based on Hippocrates.

486 Nutton. *Ancient Medicine*. New York: Routledge, 2013. P319.

69079518R00180

Made in the USA
San Bernardino, CA
11 February 2018